"If excessive worry affects the quality of your life, you owe it to yourself to get a copy of *The Worry Trick* by David Carbonell. A wise and caring teacher, Carbonell explains why the old, timeworn strategies to conquer worry don't work very well, and why our best attempts to get rid of worry end up falling flat. In *The Worry Trick*, Carbonell teaches strategies that will most likely be new to you, and work amazingly well. Writing in a style that is both entertaining and easy to understand, Carbonell uses his wry sense of humor to great advantage. As I read the book, I marked many sections that provided valuable tools and insights, and others that made me smile or laugh out loud. I especially liked his comment that our strong-willed attempts to 'stop worrying' are like 'trying to grab a greased pig on ice!' So, if worry is affecting your life, don't miss out on the solutions—and yes, *the fun*—you will find in *The Worry Trick*."

—**Neal Sideman**, self-help advocate, internationally known
coach and teacher for people recovering from anxiety
disorder, member of the Anxiety and Depression Association
of America (ADAA), and former cochair of the ADAA
Public Education Committee

"Finally, someone has written a book about worry that I can give to my clients that I'm certain will be helpful to them as they struggle to better understand and deal with their constant worrying. So very many of my clients worry constantly and have searched in vain for tools and techniques to help them, but now Dave Carbonell has given them what they were looking for—a treasure chest of tips and ideas for handling worry. This is an eminently readable book that I'm sure I will recommend to many of my clients for years to come."

—**Robert W. McLellarn, PhD**, founder and director of the
Anxiety and Panic Treatment Center, LLC, in Portland, OR

"This is the best book on worry I have read. It has all you need to put an end to ongoing, painful, toxic worry. Carbonell speaks in a clear, witty, no-nonsense style, and explains why you have been unable to contain worry so far. He gives a comprehensive explanation of why the worry trick has fooled you into inadvertently keeping worry alive, even when you are trying so hard to make it go away. Read this book if you are a worrier, if you want to help a loved one who is a worrier, or if you are a professional treating a worrying client. There is no magic cure for ending worry—it takes effort and a good bit of courage, and it is easy to lose your way. This book is a flawless road map."

—**Martin Seif, PhD**, founder of the Anxiety and
Depression Association of America (ADAA), associate
director at the Anxiety and Phobia Treatment Center
at White Plains Hospital, creator of Freedom to Fly,
and coauthor of *What Every Therapist Needs to Know
About Anxiety Disorders*

"Thank you, Dave, for writing such a treasure of a book for those struggling with anxiety and out-of-control worry. Worry has a way of convincing those experiencing it that it is VERY SERIOUS and IMPORTANT and must be immediately attended to. The key to freeing oneself from worry is learning how to relate to it from a new perspective. This fabulous book, *The Worry Trick*, teaches readers how to move past worry by offering simple, easy-to-implement techniques. I plan on recommending it to all of my clients who struggle with uncomfortable, out-of-control worrying."

—**Debra Kissen, PhD, MHSA**, clinical director at
Light on Anxiety Treatment Center, and coauthor
of *The Panic Workbook for Teens*

"Have you ever thought of yourself as having a relationship with worry? In *The Worry Trick*, David Carbonell turns worry into characters— Uncle Argument or even a flatworm—so that it becomes possible to figure out what to do and, most importantly, how to change that relationship. With a lively sense of humor, Carbonell offers vivid images and analogies to help readers understand and do something about changing that relationship with worry. In my work on mental skills for optimal performance with athletes, performing artists, and business executives, we often address issues of performance anxiety. After reading *The Worry Trick*, I started using many concepts with clients; it's a book that I will strongly encourage my clients to read as well."

—**Kate F. Hays, PhD, CPsych, CC-AASP**, founder of The Performing Edge in Toronto, ON, Canada; and past president of the Society for Sport, Exercise, and Performance Psychology

"No 'tricks' here! Carbonell's book is chock-full of advice based on the two leading evidence-based psychological treatments (cognitive behavioral therapy and acceptance and commitment therapy) for anxiety and worry. He presents concepts derived from these treatments in an extremely easy-to-digest manner, using imaginative metaphors and clear examples from his clinical practice to help illustrate them. This makes *The Worry Trick* an excellent option—either as a stand-alone resource or as an adjunct to treatment—for people struggling with chronic worry, as well as for providers interested in broadening their knowledge and skills at treating it."

—**Simon A. Rego, PsyD, ABPP, ACT**, director of psychology training and the cognitive behavioral therapy (CBT) training program at Montefiore Medical Center, and associate professor of clinical psychiatry and behavioral sciences at Albert Einstein College of Medicine in New York, NY

"Highly accessible with a minimum of jargon and 'psychobabble,' Carbonell's new book will benefit worriers of all stripes—from occasional ruminators to chronically anxious individuals with obsessive-compulsive disorder (OCD) or social, illness, or generalized anxiety disorder (GAD). *The Worry Trick* is written in an engaging, conversational style with abundant compassion and a terrific sense of humor. The author uses clever analogies and metaphors to simplify and bring to life scientifically based psychological concepts and interventions. His tone reflects decades of clinical experience helping anxious people build coping skills to achieve a more balanced perspective of their lives. *The Worry Trick* bridges the gap between more traditional cognitive behavioral therapy (CBT) for anxiety disorders and cutting-edge acceptance-based methods. I will be recommending it to hundreds of patients in my practice."

> —**David J. Kosins, PhD**, licensed psychologist in Seattle, WA; clinical instructor in the departments of psychiatry and psychology at the University of Washington; and founding fellow and certified trainer/consultant at the Academy of Cognitive Therapy; with thirty-plus years in private practice, focusing on CBT for anxiety disorders

"Dave Carbonell's clear emphasis on theory and techniques to address *worry as process* has made a profound difference in my work with anxious clients. His witty and wise approach provides specific interventions that a therapist can apply immediately—while avoiding the trap of running in circles when we try to challenge the content of our clients' worry themes."

> —**Carl Robbins, MS, MEd, LCPC**, director of training at the Anxiety and Stress Disorders Institute of Maryland, approved licensed clinical professional counselor (LCPC) supervisor, and clinical instructor in the department of psychiatry at the University of Maryland School of Medicine

"I would recommend this book to all the patients at our center. Reading *The Worry Trick* will bring welcome education and direction to anyone experiencing anxiety and worry. Carbonell's voice is concrete and calming in providing helpful information and practical strategies. It's as if the reader is one of his patients, sitting together in a group in his office. His approach is clear, compassionate, and current. To read his book is to know how the anxious mind works and how one can work toward, and achieve, a life of liberation from worry. Wonderfully clear, wonderfully understandable—*The Worry Trick* is an encouraging and useful guide for helping readers sort through the complexities of their worried minds."

>—**Judy Lake Chessa, LMSW**, coordinator at the Anxiety and Phobia Treatment Center at White Plains Hospital in White Plains, NY

"Not only is Dave a friend; he is a collaborator, a fellow speaker, and he has a dry, witty sense about him. No wonder he figured out worry better than most people have—he was able to see worry for what it was—a trick that we play on ourselves to try to make everything better only to actually make everything worse. Want to learn how to deal with your own worry, or how to help your patients deal with their worry? Read this book. Want to have great examples to give to your clients or to use in your own life? Read this book. Want to finally smile and laugh again? Do what Dave advises you to do."

>—**Patrick B. McGrath, PhD**, clinical director of the Center for Anxiety and Obsessive Compulsive Disorders (OCD) at Alexian Brothers Behavioral Health Hospital

THE
WORRY TRICK

How Your Brain Tricks You
into Expecting the Worst and
What You Can Do About It

David A.
Carbonell, PhD

New Harbinger Publications, Inc.

Publisher's Note

Distributed in Canada by Raincoast Books

Copyright © 2016 by David A. Carbonell
New Harbinger Publications, Inc.
5674 Shattuck Avenue
Oakland, CA 94609
www.newharbinger.com

Cover design by Amy Shoup
Acquired by Melissa Kirk
Edited by Christine Sabooni

Library of Congress Cataloging-in-Publication Data

Names: Carbonell, David A., author.
Title: The worry trick : how your brain tricks you into expecting the worst and what you can do about it / David A. Carbonell.
Description: Oakland, CA : New Harbinger Publications, Inc., [2016] | Includes bibliographical references.
Identifiers: LCCN 2015039307| ISBN 9781626253186 (pbk. : alk. paper) | ISBN 9781626253193 (pdf e-book) | ISBN 9781626253209 (epub)
Subjects: LCSH: Worry. | Anxiety--Prevention.
Classification: LCC BF575.W8 C296 2016 | DDC 152.4/6--dc23 LC record available at http://lccn.loc.gov/2015039307

Printed in the United States of America

22   21   20

15   14   13   12   11

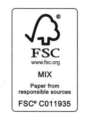
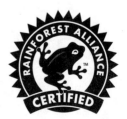

This book is for all those courageous souls who came to my office and opened my eyes to the ways of worry and anxiety. I have learned so much from you! I hope this captures some of it.

Contents

Foreword   vii

Introduction   1

1   The Worry Trick   7

2   It's All In My Head—and I Wish It Would Leave!   23

3   Your Dual Relationship with Worry   43

4   Feeling Afraid in the Absence of Danger:
How Odd Is That?   63

5   Putting Out Fires with Gasoline, and the Rule
of Opposites   79

6   The Mad Libs of Anxiety: Catch the Worries
Before They Catch You   95

7   Thinking About Thoughts   109

8   Uncle Argument and Your Relationship with Worry   125

9   AHA! Three Steps for Handling Chronic Worry   141

10   Your Daily Worry Workout   157

11   The Worry Parasite   179

12   Breaking the Secrecy Trap   191

13   Specialized Worries: Sleep and Illness   205

14   Closing Thoughts: There's Something Funny
About Worry…   225

Notes   231

Foreword

It gives me great pleasure to introduce this book. When I first got to see the manuscript, I became so excited that I wanted to start recommending it to most of my patients and virtually all the therapists I know even before it was printed. There is an ever-expanding variety of self-help books out there to choose among, but this is one that should not be overlooked. This is something radically original. There are so many little gems. Dr. Carbonell has a way of saying things that just makes you stop and reconsider long-held beliefs and practices. And who would expect that a book about worry could actually be fun to read? But chapter after chapter contains examples and descriptions of thought processes and typical absurd worry scenarios that evoke a gentle smile of recognition. The foibles of the typical anxious mind are described so astutely and so kindly that you just keep reading. And then he describes how to get out of worry loops in a way that is both counterintuitive and makes all the sense in the world.

Who should read this book? People who worry too much, people who worry about their worrying, people who love people who worry, people who treat people who worry. This book is for people who have never before considered reading a self-help book, and for people who have a stack of them on their night tables. It is for people who have never been in therapy, people who are in therapy now, and people who have tried therapy and been disappointed. Even people who have tried cognitive behavioral therapy and medication and found both somewhat helpful will find something new and liberating here.

In the history of psychotherapy, there have been many approaches to worry, all derived from the psychological theories of the day. For decades, therapy for worriers was a search for insight into "why" people were anxious about whatever they worried about, with the expectation that finding the causes of the worrying would make it melt away. But while many people learned a great deal about themselves, often the worry continued unabated. Another school of therapy suggested that since worry is essentially negative irrational thought, pointing out thinking mistakes and changing these thoughts to more rational or positive thoughts would work to relieve it. However, often people do actually know what the "right" things to think are, but the worries creep back and continue to create misery. Then people worry even more about what is wrong with them, so that they cannot listen to their own best advice during endless internal debates.

Dr. Carbonell shifts the conversation about worry from efforts to analyze or banish it to changing one's relationship to it, so that the presence of doubt or worry thoughts causes minimal distress. He puts an end to the internal fight by refusing to fight; if you refuse to dignify the contents of worry with concern and attention, you deprive your worries of what they need to grow and thrive. He illustrates how a shift in attitude can liberate joy and other emotions that have been overtaken. Worry thoughts are treated not as signals or messages or news or calls to urgent action, but as unanswerable questions not worth engaging with. Learning to distinguish between thoughts that lead to helpful action and the "nagging" of an anxious brain is the first task he teaches. From there, he takes the reader on a step-by-step journey to recovery.

Dr. Carbonell is a wise and nonjudgmental observer of the human mind, and all of us can benefit from his teachings. Having the courage to pick up this book was the first step. Take this journey at your own pace, and you will find yourself offering the book to others even before you have finished reading it.

—Sally Winston, PsyD

Introduction

Joe sits at the table, having dinner with his wife and kids. The children are excited, talking about their first day of school and everything that happened there. If you were at the table, you might notice that Joe is quieter than his wife, but he nods enthusiastically at different points and seems to be involved in the discussion.

However, if you could eavesdrop on Joe's thoughts, you'd get a very different picture. Even as he nods his head, and looks from person to person, the conversation inside his head isn't at all about the first day of school, or even about the family meal. Joe's not paying much attention to what happens now at the dining table where his family sits, out there in the "external world." Joe's mind is focused on his imagination of another place and another time, in his "internal world."

The boss comes back tomorrow, Joe's thinking, *and she's going to want to see my draft report on the marketing plan. What if she doesn't like it? What if she thinks it should be more polished by now? I'm at the top of my pay grade, what if she thinks they should go with a younger, less expensive guy?*

Joe suddenly becomes aware that his external world has become quiet. His family has stopped talking, and all eyes are on him. He shifts his attention, looking from face to face. "What is it?" he asks.

"Daddy!" his daughter shouts, laughing. "Aren't you going to pass the butter? I asked you twice!" Joe hastily passes the butter, makes a joke to cover his inattention, and his kids laugh at how absentminded their dad is. But Joe sees a concerned look cross his wife's face, and a new worry comes to mind. *What if she sees how worried I am about work? I don't want her to worry... Why can't I just sit here and have dinner?* And then, as the family turns their attention to the playful antics of their dog, Joe experiences another thought in the back of his mind and returns to his internal world: *I hope I sleep tonight, I really need the rest before I see the boss—what if I have trouble sleeping?*

Some people only experience this kind of worry infrequently, perhaps in response to a new problem in life, but this isn't an isolated instance for Joe. He has similar experiences in other situations—staff meetings; conversations with his boss; Sunday nights at home, when he's talking with his wife while watching TV, and his thoughts turn to the work week ahead; and more.

Joe worries a lot. It's not apparent to most people. In fact, he's often described by people he knows as a really calm guy. "Nothing bothers Joe!" they say. It's an act. Inside his own mind, in his internal world, Joe is often bothered, often struggling to get his thoughts to behave and stop bothering him. It rarely works.

Worry is a common and bothersome occurrence for most of humanity. What is worry?

Worries are simply thoughts and images we experience that suggest something bad about the future. Nobody knows the future, but worries pretend that they do, and that it's going to be bad, really bad.

Worries come uninvited, like party crashers. These party crashers are like fanatics on a mission. They have a message they think is important, a warning. They're going to present that warning, again and again, even though it detracts from the party atmosphere, even though no one wants to hear it, because they think they can save you from trouble this way.

Nobody enjoys the arrival of the worries. Nor do people feel grateful for the warnings, because they sense that they're overblown and unlikely, focused on hypothetical problems that probably won't happen. And yet, they're often hard to dismiss from your mind. Your attention gets turned away from your own agenda and the world around you. It gets focused on your internal world, full of thoughts about possible bad troubles, the same way that drivers turn their attention from the road to look at an accident on the shoulder.

Joe is particularly frustrated by his worry. It interferes with his enjoyment of life, invades his leisure time, and, despite the successes he has in life, leaves him feeling like a fraud.

If, like Joe, you're frequently bothered by unwanted worrisome thoughts, there's another aspect of worry to consider, and that is the kind of *relationship* you have with worry. Since you're reading this book, you've probably already thought about worry a lot, and yet it might not have occurred to you that you have a relationship with it. You do.

Your relationship with worry includes the importance you place upon your worries; how you interpret your worries; how you feel, emotionally and physically, in response to your worries; what you hope to do with your worries; the ways you try to accomplish those hopes; the ways in which your behavior influences the amount of worry you experience; the ways in which your worries influence your behavior; and the beliefs you hold about worry. In this book, I'll help you take a good look at your relationship with worry and change it to your advantage.

Probably the most important aspect of the relationship people have with worry is how worry consistently *tricks* them. If you frequently experience more worry, and more trouble with worry, than you find reasonable and ordinary, it's probably because the worry trick has shaped the relationship you have with worry in ways that make your worry more persistent and upsetting. In this book, I will help you identify the worry trick, find evidence of it in your own life, and change your relationship with worry so that its power to disrupt your life shrinks to more ordinary levels.

You might experience worry as a problem all on its own. Or you might experience worry as part of a broader problem, called an anxiety disorder, such as generalized anxiety disorder, panic disorder, social phobia, a specific phobia, or obsessive compulsive disorder. The methods I'll show you in this book can be used as a self-help method on their own or be part of a process involving the help of a professional therapist, whichever your circumstances may require.

Joe has tried hard to rid himself of his worry, with little success. It galls him when otherwise well-intentioned friends and family members suggest he simply "stop worrying," as if this were a simple problem with an obvious solution. He's tried many things—thought stopping, keeping really busy, prayer, meditation, improving his diet, exercise, nutritional supplements, seeking reassurance from his wife, seeking reassurance on the Internet, and numerous other possible solutions, with little to show for his efforts.

Still, Joe, and the millions of people like him, can reduce the disruptive effects worry has on their lives. If you find that you have more worry in your life than seems reasonable, and you have been frustrated in your efforts to reduce it, there are better ways to handle worry, and I will help you discover them and put them to work.

I suggest you use this book by starting on the first page and reading the entire book at a comfortable pace, taking notes and answering my questions along the way. I've worked with many clients who struggled with worry, and these are the methods that have been helpful to so many of them. Like them, you may feel pressured to rush through this book to get the fastest results you can. Don't do that!

A frozen pizza comes with directions like "Cook at 400 degrees for twenty minutes." If you're really hungry, or impatient, it might occur to you to think, *I'll just cook it at 800 degrees for ten minutes!* But you'll still be hungry after the fire department has left your home. Don't rush! I know you're hungry, but take your time. This book is printed in indelible ink!

The Worry Trick

This chapter will introduce you to the worry trick, and show you how people literally get tricked by their worries. This will be the first step in a process that helps you shrink the role worry plays in your life. For many people, worry is their constant, carping companion. When you come to really understand how the worry trick works, you'll get fooled less often and be much better able to reduce the worry in your life. I'm going to help you shrink worry down to an occasional nuisance.

One universal characteristic of worry is that people would like to have less of it. Nobody has ever come to my office seeking to worry more, or to have a better class of worries.

Why not? Why don't people have more appreciation for the tips and warnings that worry brings them? If thieves were stealing my car, I'd appreciate it if my neighbor tipped me off so I could call the police. I'd probably give him a reward! Why don't we feel the same way about the tips worry gives us?

Worry: An Uninvited Guest

People don't appreciate worry because it rarely, if ever, has new and useful information. Instead, it's repetition of potential problems that they're already well aware of, or warnings about possible events that are unlikely and exaggerated. It's more like nagging than news.

If worries ever had some important, useful information, you'd probably be more inclined to welcome them, but worry usually has a terrible track record for accuracy. If your worries were useful even a small percent of the time, you probably wouldn't be reading this book! Worry predictions aren't based on what's likely to happen. They're based on what would be terrible if it did happen. They're not based on probability—they're based on fear.

If worries were your neighbor, you'd move. If worries were your employee, you'd fire him. If worries were a radio station, you'd change the channel, or turn it off entirely. And therein lies the problem.

There's no off switch to your brain, and no simple way to stop the worrisome thoughts. This is what makes worry so tricky. Your natural instinct is to stop it. Of course it is! If a mosquito was buzzing near you, you'd swat it. But you don't have a good way to simply stop the worrying because we aren't built that way. It's not just that we don't have a way to stop the worry. It's much trickier than that.

Our efforts at stopping the worry almost always make things worse, rather than better.

You CAN Change Your Worry Habit

That doesn't mean you're stuck without hope of a solution. Worry is actually a manageable, workable problem. The reason people have so much trouble with worry is that worry literally tricks you. It goads you, tricks you into responding in ways that you hope will help but which actually make your troubles more severe and more persistent.

If you have struggled with worry for a long time, and find yourself unable to solve the problem, this is why. You don't have trouble solving this problem because you're too weak, too nervous, too stupid, or too defective somehow. You have trouble solving this problem because you get tricked into trying to solve it with methods that can only make the problem more severe and more chronic. I'm going to help you uncover this trick, find evidence of it in your own life, and learn how to handle worry in a more effective manner.

What Is the Worry Trick?

The trick is this: you experience *doubt*, and treat it like *danger*.

We all live our lives as if we know what's going to happen. Most days, when I leave for the office, I tell my wife and son what time I'll be home. I say it like we can count on it, but of course I don't really know for sure. I might end up booking an extra appointment and staying late; I might be home early because my last appointment cancels; I might return some phone calls that become lengthy conversations; I might have a flat tire, or get stuck in a traffic jam. If it's a really bad day, I might even die unexpectedly.

I usually don't pay much attention to those doubts. I know they're there, because I can't know what the future really holds, but they don't usually bother me too much. I just go on about my business and figure that I'll respond to events as they arise. That, literally, is life.

Danger or Discomfort?

If you or I have a doubt that really bothers us, though, we're likely to respond very differently. We're likely to treat that doubt as if it were a sign of *danger*, rather than the usual *discomfort* we can feel about uncertainty. When you get tricked into treating the discomfort of doubt as if it were danger, this leads you to struggle against the doubt, trying to remove the unwanted thoughts from your mind.

How do you struggle against the doubt? You might try hard to prove to yourself that the feared event simply won't happen. This usually results in arguing with yourself and feeling more anxious as a result. You try to "stop thinking about it," only to get the same results that come from banning books—it increases your attention to and interest in the unpleasant idea! You might try to do something to protect against the feared event and then find yourself worrying about whether or not that protection will be sufficient. You might bother your friends and family with repeated requests for reassurance. However, when they do tell you that you'll be okay, then you worry that they're just humoring you so you'll stop talking about it.

And you get dug in, deeper and deeper, with more doubt and fear, and more unsuccessful struggle against it.

Fear of the Unknown

People sometimes talk about "fear of the unknown" as if it were a special category of fear. Everything about the future is unknown! It's not the unknown part that people find scary. It's when they consider the future and think that they do know what will happen, and that it's going to be bad. That's when they get afraid.

If you were planning on cooking a special meal for your boss and her husband tonight, and experienced the thought *What if I get stuck in a traffic jam on the way home?*, you might try and remove that doubt by making sure it couldn't happen. You could set your GPS to give you notices of traffic delays; you could check the Highway Department website for notices, or call their 800 number; you could take local roads, even though that would make for a longer trip. You could call your spouse and ask what she thinks your chances are of getting stuck, trying to get some reassurance. You could develop a backup plan by identifying a restaurant that could deliver on short notice, and keep their phone number handy. That might remind you that you're very dependent on your cell phone, and you might start monitoring its battery strength very closely.

If you had a winter cold that lasted longer than usual, and experienced the thought *What if I have cancer or some other terrible illness?*, you might try similar methods to clear your mind of the worry. You might consult your physician, which is usually not a bad idea, but if that didn't clear your mind of this worry you might consult several other doctors as well. You might read up on your symptoms on various Internet sites. You might look at the obituaries, to see if anyone your age had died of cancer recently. You might look at a medical encyclopedia. You might ask the neighbors if they knew of any colds going around.

In each case, you could expend a lot of time and effort trying to prove to yourself that you have "nothing to worry about," that there is no chance of getting caught in a long traffic jam or of having cancer.

Unfortunately, you probably won't get much relief from these efforts because you can't really prove that something won't happen. You can recognize that it's very unlikely, but there's no way to *prove* to yourself that some calamity isn't going to happen tomorrow, because just about anything, no matter how improbable, is possible if your rules of evidence are loose enough.

So I can't prove that nothing will make me late for dinner tonight because it's impossible to be sure. The thought just doesn't bother me. However, if I did feel really bothered by the thought, I would probably be tempted to try to get rid of that thought, and that's where I might run into trouble.

Can You Predict the Future?

A husband who worried a lot about auto accidents would probably get very nervous whenever his wife didn't arrive home at the expected time. He might call her cell phone to verify that she was okay. And if she happened to have her phone turned off, or buried so deep in her purse that she couldn't hear it, his attempt to make himself more comfortable would result in more doubt and fear. Then he might turn on the TV, to see if there were any news stories about car crashes. He might think about calling local hospitals to see if she was there. He might drive around to see if he could spot her car somewhere, and even as he drove around, he'd worry about missing a call from the hospital on the landline (if they still have one).

He might just stay home, pacing and worrying, and wondering if he should do something.

How Worrying Backfires on You

This is a central irony of worry, that your efforts to stop worrying so often backfire on you. All too often, when you try to "talk yourself out of" a worry, you're likely to fail. Then you take your failure to prove that nothing bad will happen as evidence that something bad *will* happen. You get more worried as a result of your effort to stop worrying. That's the heart of the trick.

None of us knows the future. We know everyone dies (so far!), but we don't know when, and we don't know how. Most likely, tomorrow will be pretty similar to today. But if you try to prove it won't be different, you can't. And if you take your failure to prove that it won't be different as evidence that something bad will happen, you're in for a lot of worrying. Here's an example from my own life.

Shortly after my son was born, he developed jaundice—his skin was yellow. It's common among newborns, pretty harmless, and generally disappears within a few days. If treatment is necessary, the standard treatment is light therapy, in which the child wears a special light for several days. My son needed the light therapy.

Our conversation with our pediatrician went very poorly. My wife asked what would happen if the light didn't fix the problem. He said this was unlikely, that it almost always worked, and mentioned some really rare problems that could develop if it didn't. She asked what we could do then, and he mentioned a few minor procedures that would probably help. She asked what we'd do if those failed. The doctor said that was unlikely, but that in an extreme situation, a complete blood transfusion— the replacement of all the blood in our son's body—would probably solve the problem. She asked if that was safe, and he said that the blood supply is generally safe, but that there's always the risk of contracting AIDS, hepatitis C, and other diseases from a blood transfusion.

What an agonizing ten minutes that was! We had gone, in seconds, from arranging pretty routine care for our beautiful son, to contemplating the prospect that he would get AIDS before his first birthday. And it was all foolishness—not because we were fools, but because we all did what came naturally in our roles as parents and doctors. My wife asked for concrete answers to remote, hypothetical questions in an effort to calm her worries. The pediatrician answered them literally and completely, hoping to remove our doubts. I did nothing because I couldn't figure out how to make it better. The result was that we spent time vividly worrying about a terrible problem that was almost (but not quite) guaranteed not to happen. For several days, until the jaundice began to slowly fade, we lived with intermittent thoughts of our son contracting a dread disease.

I say "almost (but not quite) guaranteed not to happen" because you can't ever get a satisfying guarantee that something won't happen. Even if it's something that appears impossible, you won't get the certainty you want. Here's an example of what I mean.

Me: What if the law of gravity gets repealed, and we float upside down in the air, banging our heads?

Scientist: That's impossible because (insert highly technical proof), quantum mechanics, law of thermodynamics fundibulum, and blah blah blah.

Me: But what if it does happen?

Worry Always Gets the Last Word!

Let me ask you something now.

Does your car have a flat tire? (Don't look out the window!)

When I ask people this question, as we sit in my office, they almost always say no. But they can't see their car from my office. How do they know?

They don't know for sure. It's just that they didn't have a flat the last time they looked at their car, and that's good enough for them. Unless they have a particular issue of worrying about getting a flat, they assume that the tires are still okay.

But with the particular topics they worry about, they want to feel absolutely certain that they don't have a problem, and so they continually try to prove that the problem they fear doesn't, and won't ever, come to pass. If they wanted to be sure of not having a flat, they would probably want to go down to the parking lot during the session to check, and would likely mention their doubts as we talked, looking for reassurance.

There's a way out of this problem, and I've written this book to help you find it. If you're like most people who struggle with worry and anxiety, you probably have mixed feelings about even reading this book. You hope that it has some answers, but you also worry that it will create more trouble for you. You might figure that you have enough worries on your own, you don't need any help thinking up new ones! Maybe you looked at it in the bookstore and quickly scanned a few pages (or scanned some sample pages online), ready to toss it back on the shelf if you started to feel anxious reading it.

People are often so used to using distraction and other ways to try to avoid unpleasant thoughts that the idea of reading a book about worry seems worrisome! It goes against their natural instinct of seeking to avoid worry.

So you might feel more anxious when you first start to read these words. In fact, it's very likely. I understand how uncomfortable that is, but I want you to be aware that it's not a bad sign at all. The first time people come to see me for help with anxiety and worry is usually the most anxiety-provoking visit. They hope they'll get a good result, they're afraid that they won't, and they're particularly afraid that our conversation will lead them to worry more rather than less. It's anticipatory anxiety, the kind you're likely to experience just before you become engaged in a task.

Have you ever stood on a beach at the water's edge, trying to get used to the temperature of the water before you go in? You might stand there a while, feeling cold, splashing some water on your ankles, trying to get used to it, but probably feeling colder for all your effort, standing there in the breeze and feeling the difference between your skin temperature and the temperature of the water. You won't really acclimate to the water temperature until you get in it, and then you will feel more comfortable. Your natural desire to feel comfortable *first* causes you to experience more discomfort as you literally postpone and delay the moment of relief that comes with getting in the water.

That's how it usually works with worry. It's okay to feel nervous at the outset, and actually very predictable. Don't be tricked by that nervousness—it will fade. Come on in, the water's okay!

Meet the Worriers

Before I tell you any more about chronic worry, I want to introduce you to two worriers. It's a characteristic of humanity that all of us find it easier to observe and understand the patterns of other people than we do our own patterns. Perhaps hearing about other people's experience with chronic worry will help you better understand your own. In particular, having the chance to consider other people's experience with chronic worry may make it easier for you to catch on to those instances in which worry tricks you into responding in ways that make things worse.

These people don't actually exist as described below. They're composites of many, many clients I have worked with over the years. However, the details of their struggles accurately depict what it's like to wrestle with different forms of chronic worry.

Case 1: Scott

Scott sat at his desk, looking at his computer monitor and occasionally making a few keystrokes, but his mind wasn't on it. He wasn't making much progress on his report, and he worried about that. *What if I keep getting so worried that I can't work?* he worried. Visions of security personnel coming to his office to remove him and his belongings from the workplace flashed across his mind. Would his staff line up in the hallway and watch him leave? Would he go straight home and tell his wife? Would she leave him in disgust? Would he stop at a bar instead, and drink himself silly? What if he got into a drunken fight at the bar, hurt someone, and got arrested?

He noticed a headache and vaguely wondered if he was giving himself a cerebral hemorrhage with all his worrying. He wasn't sure what a cerebral hemorrhage was, or how you got one, but what if this was how it happened, sitting at your desk and worrying? He felt thirsty, and remembered some warnings he'd heard about getting dehydrated on long airplane flights. *How long is too long without water?* he wondered. Maybe dehydration contributes to cerebral hemorrhage. He pushed his chair back and got up, deciding to head for the water cooler. His back hurt. He remembered sleeping poorly last night, and hoped he'd have better luck tonight. He wondered if he'd be better off going to bed earlier, or later. What if he got so tired that he became ineffective at work?

Walking toward the water cooler, he remembered that his boss would be in all day. He'd have to pass her office on the way to the water cooler. What if she looked up and saw him walk by? What if she wondered why he wasn't in his office, working, and thought that maybe he was losing his edge? What if she called out "Hi Scott" as he was walking by, and what if he couldn't think of anything to say, and just stared or mumbled?

He had a performance review in three months. What if she took a good look at him today and realized how anxious he was? He had a long history of good work, good evaluations, and steady promotions, but what if he was topping out now, and it became obvious to her, and to everyone else? What if they had already noticed?

Scott decided he wasn't that thirsty. He went back to his office. He resumed trying to work on his report and made some revisions. But it wasn't too long before he had the thought *What if I get dehydrated and have a seizure?* He tried to distract himself by playing solitaire on his computer, but the worrisome thoughts kept breaking through. Finally, he opened his browser so he could search for information about seizures, dehydration, and cerebral hemorrhages.

And on and on it goes. Scott's actually a healthy guy, a productive and valued employee, with a good family and an apparently happy life. Scott is also a worrier.

He's tried hard to control his worry, and he's tried many things. He took medication for a while but didn't like the way it made him feel, and he worried about long-term side effects, even though the doctor said there probably wouldn't be any. He drinks more now than he used to, in an effort to fall asleep without tossing and turning. It helps him fall asleep faster, but he doesn't feel rested when he wakes, and he worries about becoming an alcoholic. He exercises and monitors his diet to keep himself as healthy as possible, but finds he's got an unhealthy mind in a healthy body. He thought about trying meditation, but was afraid of letting his mind go blank, expecting that it would get filled with more worrisome thoughts. He spends a lot of time trying to distract himself and avoiding unpleasant thoughts. He doesn't watch the news anymore, or read newspapers, because he's afraid of unpleasant topics. He avoids television shows about hospitals and other medical settings.

A Chronic Worrier

Scott's tried therapy several times, and was diagnosed with generalized anxiety disorder. He had a therapy that focused on his early childhood and life experiences; it helped him understand himself better but didn't do anything about his worrying. He had cognitive behavioral therapy, which helped him to evaluate his thoughts and find the errors in his thinking so that he could correct them; that seemed to help, but over time he found himself more focused on his thoughts, arguing with himself about whether or not a thought was exaggerated, trying to get all the "errors" out of his thoughts, feeling frustrated and apprehensive when he couldn't. He felt conflicted about writing his thoughts down and evaluating them, because sometimes it seemed to cause him more trouble, and he gradually drifted out of therapy.

Scott feels best when he's not worrying. Sometimes he'll go for days, even weeks at a time without significant worry. That feels good to him. But sooner or later, he notices how good he feels and realizes that he hasn't been worrying. And then, the thought occurs to him: *What if I start worrying again?* You can guess the rest. He resumes worrying. He tries to stop. He fails to stop, and the cycle repeats. Sometimes he's filled with despair, as he alternates between worrying about possible problems that never seem to materialize and worrying about how much worrying he does.

Scott is a chronic worrier. He has a strong case of it, but there's hope and help for him, and for you as well, if this is your burden.

Case 2: Ann

Ann worries about social encounters. She's usually okay with seeing people she already knows well but gets nervous about meeting new or unfamiliar people, encounters with bosses and people in authority, and group activities.

Ann won't go to a party or other social occasion without her husband, because she fears getting into a conversation and becoming too anxious to talk. She usually has a glass of wine, or two, before going to a social event. *What if I can't think of anything to say, and people just look at me, waiting for me to talk?* she worries. She pictures herself trapped in a social encounter, becoming visibly nervous and alarming others at the party with her excessive sweating, trembling hands, and inability to speak. As long as her husband will be with her, she figures she can ride it out because he will keep the conversation going while she calms herself or takes a bathroom break.

The idea that she could excuse herself for a bathroom break calms her a little, but she worries about that as well. She has never actually taken a bathroom break for this purpose. She has the idea that should she do so, she wouldn't be able to go back to the bathroom again during that party, because people would wonder why she was going so frequently. Since she thinks she can only do this once, like using a "get out of jail free" card in Monopoly, she figures she has to save it for emergencies, and so she really can't use it at all!

Ann feels very self-conscious about her anxiety and tries to keep it to herself. She worries what her employer and coworkers would think of her if they knew how anxious she gets about everyday conversations. Her boss has asked her on several occasions to lead a discussion at a staff meeting, and each time Ann has begged off with some excuse. She worries that she's running out of excuses. *What if my boss stops believing me?* she worries.

Fearful of Being Judged

Ann's fears have to do with being judged by people. In particular, she worries about looking so anxious that people think there's something wrong with her, avoid her, and probably gossip about her when she's not around. One of the ironies of Ann's fear is that she simultaneously believes *I am unworthy* and also *Everyone is very interested in observing and evaluating me.*

Therapy for social anxiety disorder would probably be very helpful for Ann, but she dreads the moment of sitting down with a stranger who will ask intrusive questions. *What if I start panicking right there in front of the therapist?* she worries. *I'll look like a crazy person!* The worries she has about her nervousness are what prevent her from getting the help she needs. If she can find some way to relate differently to those worries, that will be the key that enables her to move forward with her life.

Thinking It Over

Ann and Scott—and the millions they represent—have different kinds of worries, focused on different fears. What they have in common is how they relate to their worries. They struggle to bring their worries to an end and find that their worries increase rather than disappear.

"The harder I try, the worse it gets!" they notice, and feel more frustrated and incompetent as a result. They tend to think that this means they're terribly ineffective, that they can't execute a simple strategy of clearing their mind. They think it means there's something wrong *with them.*

If it's literally true—the harder I try, the worse it gets—then this probably means there's something wrong with the *methods* you've been trying. Not with you. And it means you've been looking in the wrong place if you've been blaming yourself for your worry troubles.

The very efforts people make to stop their worries are what strengthen and maintain them. Seeing how the worry trick operates in their lives—and yours—will be a valuable help in solving this problem. The next chapter will introduce you to a new way of thinking about your relationship with chronic worry.

CHAPTER 2

It's All In My Head—and I Wish It Would Leave!

If you struggle with chronic worry, there's a good chance you think you're unusual. When people come to my office for help with worry, that's usually how they think about themselves. This is a problem experienced by millions of people, all thinking they're the only one.

Everybody worries. It's part of the human condition. The only people who don't worry are dead people. Everybody experiences thoughts, generally exaggerated and unrealistic, that occur to them about bad things that could happen in the future.

I say the thoughts "occur to them" because worries aren't thoughts that you deliberately seek out. In fact, you probably try not to have them! The thoughts arise spontaneously, often against your will, or when some chance event reminds you of an unpleasant topic.

This is quite different from the deliberate thinking you do when, say, you consider buying a car. There, you consciously compare possible purchases on the basis of reliability, fuel economy, durability, safety, appearance, price, and so on. You review facts to help you make a decision. Worry is more like the intrusive comments of an annoying coworker who keeps interrupting your work with negative remarks and innuendoes that you find disturbing and unhelpful.

The Comparison Game

If you're a chronic worrier, you might think you're one of a small group because you don't see anyone who resembles your vision of yourself. Instead, you see people who seem so cool, calm, and collected that it appears they never worry, and this makes you feel inadequate by comparison.

My clients often tell me this. Seeing others who appear to be worry-free leads them to feel bad about themselves. I often feel the same way, if I'm at a party or a conference surrounded by people who seem super confident.

I usually figure I'm wrong about this, though, and if you have similar kinds of thoughts, you probably get fooled the same way I do. When you see people who appear to be cool and confident, you make this judgment from their outward physical appearance—the look on their face, their eye movements, how they hold their shoulders, the tone of their voice, their use of gestures, and so on. They look like they don't have a care in the world. You see their outer appearance and compare it to how you feel inside.

This is how you get fooled. You compare what you experience through your nerve endings to what they display on the outside. It's apples to alligators—no comparison.

What is different for some people—and this is a big difference—is how they respond to worry. That's the ball game, how you respond to it, not whether or not worrisome thoughts occur to you.

It may surprise you to hear that what you worry about, the specific content of your worrisome thoughts, isn't usually all that important. What's most important is how you relate to your worrisome thoughts, whatever their content may be.

The Content of Worries

There are differences in the content of worries and the subjects that people worry about. Some people worry mostly about ordinary events, problems that occur to most people at some point in their lives. It's common to worry about such topics in response to negative changes in life circumstances. During an economic downturn, for instance, lots of people experience thoughts about what they'd do if they lost their jobs or had trouble paying the rent or mortgage. They might have similar worries about losing their jobs or homes when there's some other change, like a new boss or landlord, which increases the uncertainty in their business relationships.

Sometimes people respond to these worries by developing a plan of action, and then the worry often fades and can be considered to have served a useful purpose. It identified a potential problem and led you to prepare a solution.

Are You an Equal Opportunity Worrier?

Other times people experience worry not in response to negative developments, but quite the opposite—they worry when good things happen!

A parent might experience worries about losing a job, even when the economy is good and his work evaluations excellent, or when a child gets accepted at his first choice of (an expensive) college and congratulations would be in order. A person leaving for a dream vacation, who's never forgotten to turn off the coffee pot and doesn't usually ever give that a thought, may be plagued by worries about that coffee pot after having boarded the plane. "Good" events, maybe a job promotion or the arrival of a new child, can often be the trigger for persistent, unrealistic worries about other possible problems in life.

People worry in response to these positive events out of a superstitious thought that now would be a particularly "bad time" for the event to occur. Thoughts such as *Wouldn't it be ironic* if the problem happened now, and *Now I have so much more to lose* are what often convert good developments into occasions for worry.

So people may experience an upsurge in worry in response to good events or bad. Worry usually has a very poor record for predicting what actually happens in the future because worry is based on ideas of what "would be bad" rather than what is likely. If worry was your stockbroker, you'd fire him!

Other times people get caught in a pattern of worrying about bad possibilities that seem far less likely, not only to most people but also to the worrier as well, at least most of the time. These are the kinds of worries that people sometimes identify as "irrational" or illogical worries. This might include worries about making some kind of mistake—leaving the stove on, accidentally pouring insecticide into the sugar bowl, driving over a pedestrian without noticing—that appears to be an extreme, unlikely, even bizarre possibility. However, the possible result of such an error seems so terrible to the worrier that he or she strives to "make sure" that it doesn't happen, and this effort to be sure becomes a chronic worry activity.

To summarize, there are differences in the kinds of content people worry about. Some people experience occasional worry about fairly ordinary problems and don't find this worry to be an ongoing problem, just an occasional nuisance they can dismiss. In fact, it often signals them to take some appropriate action and can therefore be considered to be helpful.

Others, however, have much more difficulty with worry. Sometimes people worry about ordinary possibilities but find themselves unable to dismiss those worries from their minds, and worry endlessly about fairly ordinary problems. Other times people worry about possibilities that seem extreme and unlikely, so much so that that it leads them to become chronically obsessed and preoccupied.

It's not the content of the worries themselves that distinguishes ordinary from chronic worrying. The key is how we respond to worry, how we relate to it. This is what distinguishes a person with only modest, occasional worry from a person with chronic, persistently upsetting worry. It's the relationship we establish with worry, how we try to live with it and manage it, that defines the kind of worry we have.

Let's take a look.

Ordinary Worry: A Workable Relationship

Ordinary worry is sometimes unrealistic, but the unrealistic worries come and go. They don't form a consistent pattern over time. A student may worry about a test sometimes but doesn't anticipate flunking out every time there's a quiz. An employee may worry as her annual review approaches but doesn't anticipate getting fired every time she meets with her boss.

Ordinary worry is an occasional part of your life, one that doesn't usually interfere too much with your activities. Sometimes it can help focus your attention on issues that need a solution and lead you to do some planning and problem solving. This kind of worry typically ends when you have identified a solution and taken action. That's a good thing!

Other times it doesn't particularly identify a problem and lead to a solution so much as it reflects a general state of anxiety. For instance, when you're not feeling well because of several days of the flu, or you're overtired, or you're suffering a major disappointment in work or love, you may get more caught up in worries that you would ordinarily dismiss.

The ordinary worry relationship is similar to the kind of relationship you may have with a neighbor or coworker with whom you're not closely tied. You see them but don't interact very often, probably less than once a day. When you do, you say hello and are superficially nice, but you don't have a strong emotional attachment to that person, good or bad. It doesn't ruin your day if you have a disagreement with them. It doesn't make your day if you have a nice encounter with them. They're just not that important to you.

People who have this ordinary kind of relationship with worry might get into struggles with worries, but only occasionally. They know the worries pass, so they usually don't usually spend a lot of time and energy responding to the worry. They just don't care that much about the worrisome thoughts that occasionally come and go. And, perhaps the most important distinction, they don't worry about how much they worry.

The dysfunctional relationship of chronic worry, however, is something else entirely.

Chronic Worry: A Dysfunctional Relationship

Some people get more than their share of trouble with worry. Worry becomes your constant companion rather than an occasional nuisance and can seriously degrade the quality of your life.

If you experience chronic worry, you experience an excessive amount of worry over time. Who decides how much worry is excessive? The person doing the worrying! If you feel that you have too much worry in your life and want to have less, you can probably learn to shrink the role worry plays in your life.

The most important aspect of this chronic relationship with worry, however, is not the amount of worry but the way you respond to it. This most often takes the form of an argumentative, fighting kind of relationship in which you persistently struggle to control and change your worrisome thoughts, only to find that the more you resist and oppose them, the more persistent they become. The chronic relationship with worry is one in which you really care, all too much, about the worries, and try again and again to reform them.

What Does Chronic Worry Do to You?

Chronic worry involves spending time with thoughts of possible disappointments and catastrophes, even though you don't want to. It involves a chaining of thoughts, the creation of an increasingly unlikely sequence of causes and effects which suggest that you will eventually suffer terrible catastrophes and lose your mind or your ability to function.

It's frustrating. You'd like to relax and watch that TV show, or read a book in the park. Maybe you're hoping to enjoy dinner with the family or lunch with a friend. But here come those worries again.

They seem uncontrollable! Just when you don't want them, there they are.

What if I get laid off?

What if my daughter flunks out?

What if I get sick and can't work?

What if a loved one dies?

What if the furnace conks out this winter?

What if I start screaming on the airplane?

What if I start shooting people like that crazy guy did?

What if the garage door opens by itself while I'm asleep?

What if I get cancer?

What if Joe can tell how nervous I feel?

What if I look nervous and the clerk thinks I'm a thief?

What if I pee in my pants during my presentation?

Chronic worry is likely to:

- *Be a major focus in your life for significant periods of time*

- *Direct your focus toward unlikely catastrophes*

- *Distract you from worthwhile tasks and responsibilities*

- *Interfere with your relationships with loved ones and other key people*

- *Generate obsessive thinking without leading to useful decisions*

- *Continue until something else replaces it*

- *Continue despite your recognition that you're wasting your time with worry*

- *Interfere with your participation in the present world*

- *Leave you feeling helpless, hopeless, and out of control*

People with chronic worry repeatedly think and rethink about the possibilities that concern them without coming up with new solutions or taking any effective action. There's no natural end point with chronic worry. It just drones on, continuing as if it has a life of its own.

The Struggle Is Not Just in Your Head

Chronic worry is often accompanied by physical symptoms and behaviors. This includes feeling restless, where you may find it difficult to relax and enjoy a quiet moment or a movie. You might jiggle your leg, shift frequently in your chair, crack your knuckles, sigh repeatedly, check your phone, and so on. It includes irritability, in which otherwise unimportant sounds and interruptions fill you with a startled or angry reaction. It includes muscular tension—backaches, neck aches, headaches, and more. It includes fatigue—feeling tired without apparent explanation. It includes upset stomach. It often includes trouble with sleep—either difficulty falling asleep or waking up earlier than you want.

Chronic worry doesn't alert you to problems that need solving. It interferes with problem solving. If you experience chronic worry, your attention is focused on unlikely hypothetical future disasters, rather than current situations that require a solution. Chronic worries don't get solved because there really isn't anything to solve. The worry just gets repeated until it's replaced by something else.

Chronic worry can become the focus of your life and crowd out activities that you might otherwise enjoy. Physically, you're in the present, in your usual environment. But mentally, your focus is on a dismal future of grim possibilities.

Finally, if you struggle with chronic worry, you try to stop worrying. These efforts to stop usually make things worse rather than better. It's like stories from Greek mythology in which a hero confronts a hydra, a serpent or dragon with many heads. When the hero cuts off a few heads from the hydra, several more heads grow in the place of each one.

I hate it when that happens, don't you?

Your Relationship with Worry

People who struggle with worry have several kinds of reactions. These reactions are a central part of the problem with chronic worry, and form your "relationship with worry." *The path to having less trouble with worry involves changing your relationship with worry rather than trying to change the worries themselves.*

You might be wondering how you got into a relationship with worry in the first place. Let's consider how that happens.

How Do You Get to This Point?

First, you dislike the content of the thoughts. And that's natural; the content of worry is always negative, always about bad things that might happen in the future. Nobody has ever experienced this worry: "What if I win $50 million in Super Powerball and live a dream life on Tahiti?" Nobody worries about good stuff! So you become a person who's bothered by repetitive thoughts of bad possibilities.

Second, you probably recognize—at least most of the time, when you're not so caught up in the worry—that the thoughts are unrealistic. But this doesn't help you lose the thoughts! You continue to have nagging, unwanted thoughts even though you recognize that they're unrealistic.

This can be really frustrating for most worriers. I've had many conversations with clients in which we discuss the fact that the content of their worries are kind of unrealistic. There's a technique that's part of cognitive behavioral therapy (CBT) called cognitive restructuring, in which clients are helped to review their thoughts and find "the errors of thinking" so they can change their thoughts to something more realistic. It's helpful with lots of problems but often fails to solve the problem of chronic worry. Here's a common response to the cognitive restructuring: "I know!" Not "Whew—what a relief!" but "I know!" They might be a little annoyed too, on doing that work only to discover what they already knew.

They know. They don't need me to help them discover that their worries are exaggerated and unlikely. That's why they came to see me in the first place—they were bothered by repetitive thoughts of unlikely catastrophes! So just like them, you become a person who's bothered by repetitive, unrealistic thoughts of bad possibilities and wants them to stop, and is increasingly frustrated by the fact that they don't.

Third, it may seem to you that if you keep having negative, unrealistic thoughts you don't want to have, this must mean there is something wrong with you. You have the thought that people who can't control their thoughts are "out of control" and find this a scary comment about yourself. So you become a person who's bothered by repetitive, unrealistic thoughts of bad possibilities who wants them to stop, is increasingly frustrated by the fact that they don't, and fearful that this means you're losing control of yourself.

Finally, you try hard not to have the thoughts. Maybe you do this because you hate and fear the content of the thoughts. Maybe you realize that the thoughts are unrealistic but think it's a sign of mental problems to have thoughts you can't control. In either case, you try a variety of anti-worry techniques: distraction, avoidance, thought stopping, cognitive restructuring, arguing with your thoughts, reassurance seeking, drugs and alcohol, and more. And the result, all too often, is more worry. When you struggle against your worries, you generally get more worry rather than less.

And even though you dislike the worries, you might also have some unconscious beliefs about worry, beliefs which suggest that worry helps you somehow. These beliefs can also lead you to respond in ways which keep the worries alive. We'll take a look at this in chapter 11.

So it's through a process like this that you become a person who's bothered by repetitive, unrealistic thoughts of bad possibilities and wants them to stop; who is increasingly frustrated by the fact that they don't, fearing that this means you're losing control of yourself; and who wants so desperately to get rid of the thoughts that you get caught up in a struggle to rid yourself of the thoughts—only to have more, rather than less, worry as a result.

If you've become involved with chronic worry, this is what the relationship is like, and this is the problem you need to address.

Relating to Thoughts

Worry is a way of *thinking*, and that's a big part of the problem. Modern Western culture emphasizes the role of thought in life, seeing it as the end point of billions of years of evolution. If you're like most people, you probably have lots of respect for thoughts. Especially your own thoughts! You probably give the content of your thoughts a lot of attention and credibility, even when you're having thoughts that seem exaggerated and untrue.

That leads to another part of the problem. If you're like most people, you probably tend to think you should be in control of your thoughts. You may have the idea that you should only have the thoughts you find desirable and useful and not have the thoughts that you don't want. And yet…your mind has a mind of its own. It's perfectly commonplace to have thoughts that defy your sense of control, unwanted thoughts that resist your efforts to evict them. If you've ever had a song "stuck in your head," you know what I mean.

If you're not so sure that this applies to you, take a minute now and don't think about the first pet you ever had. Put the book down, sit back, and try this for a minute.

How did you do? If you're like most people, you're probably having more recollections of that pet than you have for years.

Review Your Typical Worries

Let's take a closer look at some of your worrisome thoughts. This can help you better understand the worry process and find your way out of a chronic, conflictual relationship with worry.

Is that okay with you—to look at your worrisome thoughts and write some of them down?

You might not want to do this. Maybe you have the thought that if you write them down they will get more permanently fixed in your mind, or even be more likely to come true! Maybe you'd just like to forget them as soon as possible and enjoy the rest of your day. Maybe you think that if you write them down, this will lead you to worry even more than you already do.

Maybe you're thinking, "Dave, I bought this book to get rid of my thoughts, not to write them down! I just want to be rid of them."

But maybe this is what you usually do—try to push them away. And yet here you are, reading a book about worry. What you've tried in the past probably hasn't been all that helpful. If it had, you'd probably be doing something more enjoyable than reading (and hopefully, writing) about worry!

If your past efforts to solve this problem haven't done the job, it's probably not due to the reason you imagine—that there's something wrong with you. It's more likely to be because you got tricked into using methods that weren't so helpful. You'll probably do better with a different approach. So, if you're at all willing, experiment now with writing down a few of your typical worries so you can do a little work with them.

Put Your Worries in a Lineup

This is what you would do if you had been the victim of a crime, like a mugging or a robbery. You'd report it to the police, and they would ask you to sit down with the police artist and describe the mugger so the artist could draw him. This would help the police apprehend the perpetrator. It wouldn't be pleasant, but it would be worth doing. Sketching out some of your worries to do this review might be your first step toward changing your relationship with worry for the better. Is it worth a try?

What are some worries that bothered you recently? Write down a few of them on your favorite electronic device, or do it the old-fashioned way with pen and paper.

Take a look at the worries you wrote down, and apply this two-part test.

1. Is there a problem that exists now in the external world around you?

2. If there is, can you do something to change it now?

If you answered "yes" and "yes" to these questions, then perhaps you should put this book aside and go do something to change the problem now. If there's a significant problem now in the physical world you inhabit, and you can do something to change it now, go ahead and do that!

On the other hand, if you answered "no" and "no" (or "yes" to the first question and "no" to the second), then you're dealing with chronic worry. You're nervous, and that worrisome thought is just a symptom of being nervous.

Maybe your answer was neither "yes" nor "no" but included thoughts like these:

It's not happening right now, but what if it starts soon?

If I don't stay on guard and watch out, bad things might happen.

I hope it doesn't happen, but how can I be sure?

It probably won't happen, but it would be so awful if it did...

Isn't it possible that this might happen? I sure hope it doesn't!

If I don't worry about it, then it probably will happen.

Thoughts like these are particularly tricky. You're likely to have such thoughts when you try to persuade yourself that some dreaded event just isn't possible, that it won't and can't happen. It's very difficult to "prove a negative," to prove that something "won't happen" in the future; trying to is a losing game, a response that brings you more worry rather than less.

Cross-Examine Your Worries

This is like that moment in a courtroom drama, when a witness gives a long-winded answer to a pointed question in an attempt to avoid answering it with "yes" or "no," and the judge finally orders the witness to just answer the question. You're not on the witness stand, but it will be helpful to answer these questions with "yes" or "no."

Is there a problem that exists now in the external world around you?

If there is, can you do something to change it now?

Your brain will refer you to various "possibilities." You'll have thoughts that tell you something bad could possibly happen sometime in the future. And that's true. It's always true, whether you have thoughts about it or not. Anything is possible, bad things sometimes do happen, and nobody knows the future. But this is of little help in taking care of business now. It's more helpful to notice those thoughts and still restrict yourself to choosing "yes" or "no." And if the answer isn't "yes," then it's "no."

Do your answers include these kinds of thoughts?

- *I'll never get on the right track.*

- *I won't be able to solve this because I'll always feel depressed.*

- *I don't know what the best solution is, so I'll never solve this problem.*

- *I can't make decisions, let alone good decisions. I'm doomed to suffer.*

These thoughts misdirect and mislead you by suggesting a problem in your *internal* world. The problem they suggest is usually about your being so defective—so depressed, so insecure, so uncertain, so confused, so stupid, so whatever—that you won't be able to solve your problems and live a good life.

This is a "trickier" kind of thought—a trickier form of bait—and people very often are drawn into thinking and rethinking it, obsessing about it, feeling bad about it, and, in all kinds of ways, "stuck in their heads" about it. So if you struggle with these kinds of thoughts, consider this.

How consistent are these thoughts over time? For instance, if my dog develops a limp, or a warning light comes on in my car and stays on, my thoughts are usually consistent about these problems. I don't have some days where I think the limp or the light doesn't matter. I'm aware that both represent a problem I need to solve, and I feel concern. That concern remains with me until the problem gets fixed or goes away.

On the other hand, sometimes I have a discouraging thought that I'll never be able to finish writing this book, and I feel down and depressed about that. This thought will typically last a little while and then get replaced by something very different. For whatever reason—I get a compliment on something I wrote, or I go see a funny movie, or have a nice chat with a friend—I start thinking and feeling differently about this thought of being a terrible writer. My writing ability is the same as before, and so is my draft. Yet I feel, and think, differently about it. In other words, my thoughts about my writing ability are variable and inconsistent over time.

My thoughts about my dog's limp, or the warning light in my car, remain consistent over time until I fix the problem.

If you often experience the kind of thoughts above, thoughts that voice a general sense of despair, lack of ability, or hopelessness, ask yourself these questions:

Is this thought consistent over time? Has it been the same the last seven days, and seven weeks? Or does it change—do I sometimes feel more optimistic, sometimes realize that this thought is exaggerated? Does it go up and down like emotions do?

"Just the Facts, Ma'am"

Emotions change, frequently, and often without obvious reason. Facts don't change in the absence of new evidence. If your thought varies in this way, if it changes with your mood, then it doesn't really indicate a present problem in the external world. It indicates some unhappiness or upset within yourself, in your internal world, that varies over time—a problem in how you view and relate to your internal experiences of thoughts, emotions, and physical sensations. It might be an issue that follows you periodically, like your shadow when the light is right, but it doesn't represent a problem "out there" in the external world any more than your shadow represents an assailant. It's not a problem that you can, or must, solve right now. It's a problem that plays out in your mind, without any corresponding reality in the external world. And it's part of the burden of being human.

If you had a problem in the external world you had to solve right now, or suffer bad consequences, you'd know it, and you'd be doing something about it. If your dripping sink were stopped up and about to overflow, you'd be draining, not worrying. If your dog were whining and looking at the door, you'd be walking, not worrying.

Odds are, if you're experiencing chronic worry right now, you don't have a real problem in the external world. In fact, if the sink overflowed right now, or the dog started frantically scratching at the door, you'd probably quickly shift gears and take care of the problem. Worrying would be gone, for the moment.

Feelings vs. Thoughts

Sometimes people mistake feelings for thoughts. For instance, you might hear someone say, "I feel like I'll never get a good job" or "I feel like I'm in danger." But these aren't feelings. They're thoughts. Thoughts are ideas. Feelings are emotions, and they're quite different from thoughts. Thoughts can be true or false, or somewhere in between. Feelings are emotional responses that don't involve true or false. So when we look at these two examples, I think they're more accurately put like this:

I think I'll never get a good job, and I feel sad about that.

I think I'm in danger, and I feel fear about that.

The thoughts—about never getting a good job or about being in danger—may be true or false. The emotions are reactions to the content of the thoughts, regardless of how true or false that content is. We can experience an emotional response to a false thought just as powerfully as we can to a true thought. Our emotions are reactions to the content of our thoughts, regardless of the reality (or lack thereof) behind the thoughts.

This realization, that we can have strong emotional responses to thoughts that are false as well as those that are true, is the basis for doing cognitive restructuring, which aims at making our thoughts more realistic. It can often be helpful. However, it's common for people who are stuck in chronic worry to find cognitive restructuring, and other efforts to edit their thoughts into more realistic versions, somewhat less helpful than they hoped. We'll take a look at that problem in the next chapter.

Thinking It Over

Worry is common, a universal part of the human experience, but because it's not generally visible to others, you're likely to think that you're one of a very few, maybe the only chronic worrier in the world. Not so!

What you worry about isn't nearly as important as how you relate to the worry, how you try to get it under your control. The path out of chronic worry will take you into an examination of how you deal with worry. It's there that you are likely to find that you've been using methods to control worry that are akin to cutting heads off the hydra—it just leads to more heads that bite and breathe fire! Recovery from chronic worry will involve replacing those methods with something more effective and thereby changing your relationship with worry.

We'll take a more detailed look at your responses to worry in the next chapter.

CHAPTER 3

Your Dual Relationship with Worry

When I was training to become a psychologist, I had my first experience working with a client who struggled with worry. This man worried a lot about losing his job. He obsessed over every tiny error or shortcoming he displayed at work and overlooked all his good accomplishments on the job. My supervisor wanted me to learn to use cognitive restructuring with this client, which, you may recall, is a method by which people can find and correct the "errors" in their thinking that cause distress.

The supervisor expected me to become good with these techniques, so I worked hard at it. I helped my client become aware of how he was "maximizing" all the negatives in his mind and "minimizing" all the positives so that his job seemed less secure than it probably was. And one day, we had a session in which the man seemed to show some good progress. "I see what you mean," he told me. "I've been overlooking all the good things I do at work, and overemphasizing the things that can use some improvement. My boss seems okay with the idea that I need more experience and training, and he seems happy with most of the results I get even though I'm new. So I guess I've really been exaggerating the risk of getting fired."

I smiled, happy for his progress, and looking forward to describing it to my supervisor. Then he continued, once again getting upset, "So you see, that's what really worries me. Look at all the unnecessary worry I've been doing! That can't be good for my health! What if it gives me a stroke, all this worrying about nothing?"

My heart sank as I realized we hadn't made as much progress as I thought! But I should really thank this man, if he happens to be reading this book, for giving me such a clear example of the two stances of the worry relationship. On the one hand, he took the thought about losing his job very seriously and worried intensely about it. On the other, when he realized that this worry was unrealistic, he worried about how much worrying he was doing! And, when I saw him the following week, he had thought of some more reasons to believe that he might get fired and was back to worrying about that. He was treating these thoughts the way you might respond to a piece of cactus stuck in your hand—too painful to leave alone and too painful to remove!

This man—and most people who struggle with chronic worry—didn't have a problem that he worried about. He had the problem of worrying.

The Two-Sided Relationship with Worry

If you struggle with chronic worry, odds are that you associate the worries with danger, in two ways.

Sometimes, you take the content of the worry thought as an important prediction of danger. It might seem to you that thoughts such as *What if I lose my job?* or *What if I have cancer?*

are valid warnings about trouble with your employment or your health, a sign of trouble in your external world. In response, you either try to protect against that hypothetical danger or you try to prove that there isn't any danger, so that you can feel better and stop worrying.

Both of those responses tend to fail.

Other times, you recognize that these thoughts are "irrational" or unlikely, and you don't take the content of the worry so seriously. Instead, you wonder why you keep having such grim and unlikely thoughts. You might take the presence of the thought as a sign that something is going terribly wrong in your mind, in your internal world. You may think that you shouldn't have such thoughts at all, that the thoughts themselves are a sign of you losing control of yourself. You might fear that such thoughts might even make you ill. In response, you try in various ways to suppress or rid yourself of the thought.

This response also tends to fail.

Your relationship with worry may take two different forms. Let's take a closer look at how each one works.

Stance 1: Treat the Worry as an Important Warning

This is the first stance. You take the content of your worry seriously, and:

1. Look for ways to disprove the threats, and reassure yourself that the feared catastrophes won't come to pass; and/or you

2. Think of ways you could protect against the feared events, and either use them or "keep them in mind" as a future defense.

People will frequently take both steps above, even though, if you could prove an event wasn't going to happen, you wouldn't need to defend against it. So a person having thoughts of getting sick and missing work might try to soothe himself this way: "I won't get sick, I had a flu shot, and anyway I have lots of sick time left over."

Let's look at some of the common ways people use this stance.

Arguing with the Worry

You might get into a debate with your own thoughts, the same way you might if you were arguing with another person. It's a game of "point-counterpoint" and often sounds like this.

Me: What if I lose my job and we all end up on the street?

Also Me: That's not going to happen—they need me at the firm!

Me: What if it does?

No matter what evidence or ideas you bring to the argument to reassure yourself, the other side of the debate always has a strategy for topping your argument, as we see here.

Also Me: It's really unlikely I'm going to lose my job, but if I do, I'll just find another one. We'd get by.

Me: But what if you don't?

This "what if" argument is a central part of chronic worry, and we'll take a good look at how it works, and what to do about it, in chapter 6.

These debates you have with yourself are really circular. When you're debating these worries, do you bring in any new evidence since you last had the debate?

Probably not! Instead, you find yourself repeating the same tired old points, having pretty much the same debate each time. The same thoughts keep getting repeated, again and again, without any progress, new ideas, or problem solving. No wonder it gets so annoying! If it were a television program, you'd turn it off or change the channel—but this TV set doesn't have any controls!

If you find yourself arguing with yourself, there's one thing you can count on—you're not going to win this argument.

How does the debate end? There's no real conclusion. It ends when your attention is drawn to something else. Given how tedious this ongoing repetition of worries can become, it's no wonder you lose interest!

But it'll probably be back, same as before, the next time your mind is idle.

Ritualistic Responses

You might take this a step further and engage in private, subtle behaviors you hope will end the debate. So a person who worries about choking and gagging may continually drink small amounts of water, either hoping to keep his throat "open" this way or trying to prove that there isn't any problem. A person who worries about leaving the stove or coffee pot on might linger in the kitchen before going to work, playing with the on-off switch, or even unplug it. A person who fears dying in a plane crash may touch the skin of the airplane while boarding, "just for luck."

These responses are a lot like superstitions.

Here are some common ones.

- *Singing or humming a song to yourself*

- *Praying with the expectation of a clear, reassuring answer from God (preferably in writing!)*

- *Thinking about other people's problems and telling yourself to be grateful*

- *Snapping your fingers*

- *Putting your worries in a "worry jar" or something similar*

- *Relying on luck—your lucky shirt, lucky breakfast, and so on*

- *Counting something—the number of letters in a word; the number of words in a sentence; the number of people in line; the total of the numbers in a license plate*

People generally recognize that such responses won't really alter anything in the external world, but they continue to use them, perhaps with the thought, *It can't hurt!* If you use them occasionally, with a sense of humor and without ascribing any real power to them, they probably won't hurt your cause. However, if you find yourself in a pattern wherein you feel more nervous if you refrain from your ritual, and feel as though you "must" follow this habit, then it probably *does* hurt.

Internet Research (Googling)

The Internet has opened up new frontiers for people who struggle with worry. Before there was an Internet, you had to visit a library or a bookstore to research your worries. Now, with the click of a mouse, anyone with fingers can enter a couple of search terms and see what comes back.

The irony is that people do this hoping to find out that they have nothing to worry about. So if you're a person who worries that your cough might be a sign of cancer, or that your garage door opener might be set off by someone's microwave, you might go to the web hoping to find a page that says it's not so. This might work—there's a chance that you'll find some web pages with useful information for you.

However, if you want to eliminate all doubt, if you're hoping to find conclusive evidence that proves you don't have cancer or your garage door can't ever open by accident, you're likely to be disappointed. As much as you might like to get absolute proof that this problem isn't occurring now, and can't ever occur in the future, that evidence is not available, because we can't prove that something will never happen. When you struggle mightily to feel sure, it's like you're hoping to find a web page with your photo and name on it, and a message saying that you're guaranteed to be okay. That page is not available! Even if it were, that wouldn't be the end of it. If you ever did find such a page, you'd probably find yourself wondering, "How can they be so sure?"

Consult Experts

This comes up most frequently about health concerns, but people with other types of worries—about finances, real estate, taxes, child rearing, career planning, and so on—also get caught up in this.

If you consult an expert about a worry—maybe a cardiologist about your heart, or an accountant about your taxes—a consultation with one expert should generally be enough. In some cases, with really complex issues, maybe a second opinion will seem necessary. But if you find that you get caught in a pattern of seeing a variety of professionals about your concern, and remain too doubtful to actually use any of the recommendations—if you come away from the consultations with more questions or hypothetical reasons to distrust the answers you received—then you're probably caught up in a cycle of seeking more and more professional reassurance, and feeling less and less sure as a result.

Consult "Non-Experts"—Friends, Family, Coworkers, and Neighbors

In addition to, or often in place of, consulting experts, worriers frequently ask loved ones, relatives, friends, and coworkers for reassurance. They don't ask these people for reassurance because they have some special expertise or knowledge of the topic. They ask these people because it's convenient and free!

Because of this, they put even less confidence in the reassurance they receive from these "civilians" than they do in the expert opinions they received. The discussions they have with family or friends often devolve into something like the argument they have in their heads, with the worrier trying to find flaws in the reassurance being offered. They wonder if the other person is just saying what they want to hear, or humoring them to get them to change the topic. If you engage in this pattern, you probably don't ask just once. You might ask repeatedly, asking the question in different ways to see if you get the same answer. Reassurance has a very short shelf life and lasts only a little while before you start seeking a fresh supply.

This kind of reassurance seeking can be a burden on a marriage, friendship, or other relationship. The party being asked for reassurance often becomes increasingly concerned that he or she doesn't really know what's helpful to do—to continue to answer the questions or "call the question" and encourage the asker to find his own answers.

Avoidance

Another way that people take their worries seriously is with the use of avoidance. It's very common for people to avoid what they fear, even when they recognize that their fears are exaggerated or unrealistic, and even when the avoidance comes with a significant disadvantage.

You might avoid conversations with your boss, even though such contacts might help your career and facilitate your work. You might avoid group activities where you fear being observed and judged, like open house at your children's school or a neighborhood block party, even though this limits your social life; you might avoid answering the phone, or making calls; you might avoid going for your annual physical; you might avoid a task because you feel compelled to do it perfectly and worry you'll have trouble finishing it. You might avoid certain locations or activities for fear of having a panic attack there.

If you fear public speaking, you're likely to avoid requests to address a group, be it at work, your child's school, or a civic organization. If you fear plane crashes, even if you are familiar with the safety statistics showing that flying is the safest form of travel, you're likely to avoid flying or endure it with great discomfort and the use of alcohol or tranquilizers. Highway driving, dogs, elevators, being alone, sitting in the middle of a pew—if you worry about it, there's a good chance you avoid it.

This is a real problem when you yourself recognize that your worry is based on an "irrational" fear. "I know it doesn't make any sense," people say. "That's what really bothers me about these thoughts!"

Your recognition that your worries are exaggerated or unrealistic doesn't help you if you continue to avoid what you fear anyway. If you avoid the object of your worries, you will become more afraid of them. What you do counts for much more than what you think.

Cognitive Restructuring Taken Too Far

If you've ever worked with a cognitive behavioral therapist, or read any self-help books based on cognitive behavioral therapy, you've probably tried cognitive restructuring. When you do cognitive restructuring, you identify the mistaken thoughts that fuel your upset and replace them with thoughts that are more realistic. Then, hopefully, you are less bothered by these new thoughts.

Proponents of cognitive restructuring have identified a number of these "errors of thinking" in order to help people identify and change them. These include such errors as:

Overgeneralizing—*believing that one bad moment means the whole day is going to be terrible*

Mind reading—*thinking you can tell what others are thinking, especially about you*

Maximizing *bad probabilities and* **Minimizing** *your ability to adapt to difficulties*

Fortune telling—*thinking you know what the future holds*

Black and white thinking—*thinking of extremes without recognizing the middle ground*

Cognitive restructuring can be very helpful with a variety of problems. For instance, a speaker who gets nervous on seeing people in the audience who yawn or look at their watches probably has some thoughts to the effect that they do this because he's boring, and that's why he feels nervous. However, if the speaker can review these thoughts and recognize that there are many reasons why audience members might do such things—they didn't sleep well, they have to leave early for another meeting, and so on—then he might become more accepting of their yawns and watch checking without necessarily taking such behaviors as negative comments on the quality of his presentation.

However, it's likely to cause you more trouble if you use it in an effort to *abolish* your bad thoughts, and become "sure" that your worries will not come true. This is where you might find yourself crossing over into the second stance. A successful public speaker might still experience the same thoughts as a nervous one when she observes yawns during her presentation and just not pay them any mind, treating them like background noise while she goes on with her talk. However, if a speaker tries to eliminate these thoughts from her mind, on the grounds that the thoughts are mistaken and should not present themselves, then she's likely to end up talking more to her worries than to her audience. In this case, cognitive restructuring may work just like arguing with your worry and bring you back to the original problem.

If you want to use cognitive restructuring, be guided by the results you get. If you find that these methods help you recognize that your worries are exaggerated and unrealistic, and you become less bothered by them, then you're getting good results and can expect to continue to benefit from using them. However, if you find that your efforts to identify and remove the "errors" in your thinking lead you to argue more with your thoughts in an effort to remove all uncertainty, then you're probably trying too hard to purify your thoughts. It might help to do the cognitive restructuring with a lighter, more permissive touch. (It might also help to use some of the acceptance-based methods I'll introduce in chapters 8 to 10 in place of cognitive restructuring.)

Now let's look at the other stance in this dual relationship with worry.

Stance 2: Stop Thinking That!

People take this stance when they become worried about how much worrying they're doing. In Stance 1, they were very concerned about the potential problems they were thinking of, but now it seems clear to them that the thoughts are just a bunch of worthless worry, of noisy nonsense. Unfortunately, this doesn't lead them to feel any better. Instead, they worry about doing so much worrying! They start having thoughts like, *These thoughts don't make any sense, why can't I stop them? What if I get a heart attack or stroke from all this worry?* or *What if these thoughts prevent me from doing my job and I get fired?* or *Why do I worry so much? I must be going crazy!*

When you experience these kinds of thoughts, you're on the other side of the worry street. You're not trying to disprove the thoughts. In fact, you might be quite clear that the thoughts are "irrational" and not to be believed. That's good. Unfortunately, though, you're now in a different kind of struggle—the struggle to "stop worrying."

With Stance 1, you were afraid that the worries were accurate predictions of trouble, and you spent a lot of time thinking about them, researching the problem, discussing it with loved ones, trying to persuade yourself that you were safe. Now, you're much less concerned with the apparent content of the thoughts. Now you're bothered by how much worrying you do, and afraid of how the worry itself might affect you. You have thoughts that worry might prevent you from ever enjoying your life, from being a good parent or spouse, that it might make you less productive at work, that it might become obvious to others and damage your reputation, even that it might literally kill you. So now you try to get the worry out of your head. You try distraction, thought stopping, avoiding the subject, anything to "stop thinking about it."

While there is some overlap, most of the ways that people try to control Stance 2 worry are different from the methods they tried with Stance 1. Here are some of the key ways people try to "stop worrying."

Distracting Yourself

A very common response is to try to distract yourself, so you don't think about the topics that worry you. Distraction sometimes works to take your mind off a problem, especially when the distraction is an outside event like an unexpected phone call, a household emergency, or your dog barking. However, you can't count on this kind of distraction—it's unpredictable and unreliable. So many people try to deliberately distract themselves from their unpleasant thoughts and worries. They might hum a favorite tune, look over some text messages they've already read, or phone a friend just to chat. This quickly becomes a source of trouble, for two reasons.

The first is that when you try to deliberately distract yourself, you're aware of what you don't want to think of. You tell yourself to "think about this, not that." Once you've done this, it's too late—you're already thinking of what you hoped to avoid!

The second reason is that the use of distraction strengthens the belief that thoughts can be dangerous. On those occasions when it works, you are literally training your mind to expect relief when the thought leaves—and therefore to feel upset when the thought remains, or returns. The more effort you make to get those thoughts out of your head, the more your mind will justify the effort by viewing the thoughts as dangerous. The truth is, thoughts simply aren't dangerous. Actions can be dangerous; thoughts can only be unpleasant. If thoughts were dangerous, the obituary pages would be banned. There's no such thing as a "killer joke." The more you use distraction, the more you strengthen this impression that thoughts can be hazardous.

A variation on distraction is when people try really hard to "think positive." It's probably a good thing to enjoy positive thoughts. But when you struggle to make your thoughts positive, all too often you're going to end up with the opposite result.

Thought Stopping

When people find their ability to distract themselves erodes over time, they often escalate their effort to *thought stopping*. Here, by sheer power of will, people sternly instruct themselves to "Stop thinking about that." They may even snap a rubber band on their wrist and say "Stop!" I'm sorry to say that this technique has actually made its way into the self-help literature, and even today you may find books advocating this technique. It ranks high among the worst advice I have ever seen in print!

Thought stopping works like banning books—it just promotes interest in the forbidden topic! It leads, inevitably, to the return of the thoughts you were trying to stop. All you'll have to show for it will be some red welts on your wrist.

Should you use thought stopping? Don't even think about thought stopping!

Use of Substances

It's quite common for people to try to control their worry with the use of substances that they ingest. Here the aim is not to dispute or contradict the content of the worries. It's simply to stop the worry thoughts from arising.

Drugs and Alcohol

People will frequently turn to the use of street drugs and alcohol in an effort to relax and quiet their mind. It works, until it doesn't, and then you have a much bigger problem than you had before.

On a daily basis, you might find that while your drug of choice helped you relax the night before, it leaves you feeling less comfortable and more anxious the next day, a hangover effect. This is part of a terrible chain of dependency in which you can become more and more reliant on the drug or on alcohol and develop the additional problem of substance abuse as a result. There isn't any problem that can't be made worse by the use of drugs and alcohol as a solution.

Tobacco use follows the same pattern.

Prescription Medications

I'm usually skeptical about the use of prescription medications for reducing worry. I think it often causes more trouble than good. It strengthens the idea that you need protection from your thoughts, and often produces unwelcome side effects.

However, I have seen the occasional client who benefited from medication when nothing else helped much. If you are going to try these medications to tame really persistent worries, be guided by the results you get. If, on balance, your life seems to work better with the medication than without, that sounds like a reasonably good use of medication.

Comfort Foods

If only the comfort lasted without adding weight, and strengthening the urge to eat! Of course it doesn't, and in this regard the reliance on emotional eating resembles the reliance on drugs and alcohol.

Avoidance of Cues and Reminders

When you're in the stance of taking your worries seriously, you may avoid situations and objects in the "real world." A person who fears flying will avoid airplanes, and similarly with people who fear dogs, driving, and so on.

When you're in the stance of simply worrying about how much you worry, you may find yourself avoiding sources of information in an effort to control or limit what you think about. You might limit your use of mass media—newspapers, television, and so on—for fear of hearing a story that triggers you to think about feared subjects. You might limit your TV watching to the Disney Channel, or your reading of periodicals to the children's *Highlights* magazine in your dentist's office (unless you fear dentists...).

In a similar way, you may hope, or expect, a spouse or friend to stop mentioning the topics you find scary, and become upset with them when they don't do a good job of this.

Like other efforts to control or limit your thoughts, these efforts usually lead people to feel more vulnerable and "on guard" rather than more comfortable and secure.

Support People

We all naturally enjoy contact and communication with others. However, sometimes people who struggle with chronic worry become dependent on one particular person for ongoing reassurance. Relying on a support person carries some of the same advantages and disadvantages as the use of alcohol to self-medicate. You can get some quick temporary relief, faster than you would otherwise; but the long-term disadvantages greatly outweigh the temporary advantage. The long-term disadvantages of relying on a support person include diminished self-confidence, as you attribute all your coping to the support person, rather than yourself, and the loss of independence and initiative, as you come to rely on and require the aid of the support person.

Support people may be pressed into service in both parts of the relationship people have with worry. In Stance 1, when you take the apparent content of the worry seriously, you may look for repeated reassurance that the feared events will not occur. In Stance 2, when you struggle to "stop thinking" about the worry topic, you might be more likely to look to the support person as a source of distraction, or a source of general reassurance that all will be well.

Does this person have any special powers? No. Their influence stems from the relationship they have with you.

Support Objects

Support objects work the same way as support people, but without the possibility of back talk. It's quite common for people to fall into the habit of carrying objects with them in an effort to reduce their worry. Sometimes these objects seem to have some logical but misleading connection to the worry, as when a person who worries about choking keeps a water bottle handy at all times. Other times they're more like a superstitious lucky charm.

While the use of such objects in an effort to reduce worry can seem harmless enough, it can cause you some problems.

You can come to believe that you need these objects to get along, and continue to feel vulnerable to worry because you suppose these objects are somehow protecting you. If you believe an object is protecting you, you'll probably worry about having an adequate supply of the object. For instance, if you have the thought that you need a water bottle to stay alive, is one bottle really enough? Additionally, while reliance on these objects may help you get some quick temporary comfort, it also prevents you from noticing that things are okay with or without the support object.

I'm reaching back into the distant past for this reference, but if you've seen the Disney movie *Dumbo* (1941), you might recognize Dumbo's feather as a support object. Dumbo, the flying elephant, mistakenly attributed his ability to fly to a magical feather, and it wasn't until he dropped the feather that he came to realize that he was stronger and more capable than he realized. You youngsters can Google it!

Here are some common support objects.

Snack foods

Pictures of grandkids or other loved ones

Books about anxiety

Cell phones

Water bottles

Items that grant "luck," like a four-leaf clover or a rabbit's foot

Worry beads

Rosary beads

Medications

Medications can be support objects independent of their medicinal effect. Many people carry Xanax and similar medications for years without ever ingesting a pill. They get relief just from knowing the bottle is in their pocket or purse! I worked with a client who worried a lot about having a panic attack, a man who enjoyed scuba diving. When he went diving, he kept a Xanax tablet strapped to his leg, in a waterproof container beneath his wet suit, even though it would be impossible to reach it during a dive!

Take Inventory

Which of the anti-worry behaviors described in this chapter do you use most frequently? Do they serve you well, or poorly? Which would you like to leave behind?

Before you move on, take a few minutes to make a list of them, and periodically review it, updating it as necessary.

Thinking It Over

In this chapter, I've described the dual relationship people establish with worry. Sometimes you take the apparent content of the worry thoughts seriously, and try to protect against the thoughts or disprove them. Sometimes you recognize that the thoughts are exaggerated and unrealistic, worry about how much worrying you do, and try hard to stop having such thoughts.

Neither response works over time. Neither is capable of giving you the relief you seek. Instead, both make your situation with worry worse rather than better and add to your sense of being "stuck" in your worries. Perhaps even worse, they may lead to the demoralizing observation "The harder I try, the worse it gets" and leave you feeling unable to help yourself.

Fortunately, there is an effective way out of this logjam. Your situation with worry has been getting worse because you're been tricked into trying things that *do* make it worse. As you come to discover this, you can turn your attention and energy to different kinds of responses to worry, responses that will reward your efforts by making your situation better. In later chapters, I will show you some methods you can try, methods which will probably bring you more of the results you want.

Feeling Afraid in the Absence of Danger: How Odd Is That?

You're probably reading this book because you're bothered by a lot of worry that you recognize is unrealistic and exaggerated. It sounds odd to say, but that's the good news. You don't really have all the problems that your worries suggest. The bad news is that these worries function like a red flag to a bull. The red flag isn't a threat to the bull, but its appearance leads the bull to charge and make himself vulnerable to the swords and spears of the matador. Your worries aren't a threat to you, but their appearance invites you to struggle to get rid of them, and that's what makes you vulnerable to more worrying. When you resist your thoughts, you hope to be the matador, but you're actually the bull.

This chapter will help you see how this kind of worry is not evidence of a weak or troubled mind but a natural consequence of how our brains are organized. This is really important, because if you keep getting "suckered" by the idea that your worries mean there's something wrong with you, you will keep getting tricked into responding in ways that make things worse, rather than better. You'll keep taking the bait. So let me show you how these worries are the natural consequence of the kind of brains we have and the world we live in. This will put you in a good position to use the different responses to worry that will come in the following chapters.

Fear for Sale

If you frequently get anxious in response to your worry thoughts—if you frequently get afraid when you're not in danger—does this mean there's something wrong with you?

The short answer is no. This is part of what it is to be human. We can feel afraid even when we *know* we're not in danger.

For evidence, you need only go to your library, your favorite bookseller, or the movie listings in your area. What's the evidence? It's the scary books and movies that are so commercially successful in our culture. Billions of dollars change hands around the globe every year in the business of scary entertainment.

You might wonder why someone would want such an experience, much less pay good money for it. That's a good question, but it's not what I find most interesting about scary entertainment. The most interesting thing about scary books and movies is that *they work*. People can read or watch material they know to be pure fiction and actually feel afraid! Scary movies may not be your cup of tea, and you certainly don't need to go see any, but I want to point out to you that they work, and to help you see what this says about humanity in general.

It's Only a Movie, But It Can Still Scare You

People who watch scary movies already know "it's only a movie." That doesn't matter. They become afraid anyway. This ability, to become afraid even when we know we're not in danger, is a characteristic of our species. If it weren't, Stephen King would be writing for *Good Housekeeping Magazine*! If you tend to blame and criticize yourself for becoming afraid of your own exaggerated and unrealistic worries, this is very important information to consider.

If you watch a really scary movie and become afraid, you might try telling yourself "it's only a movie," but this rarely takes away the fear. If you're really worried about something, and a good friend tells you to "stop worrying about that," that usually doesn't help either.

One reason this rarely works is that we don't directly control our thoughts. We can direct our attention to a particular problem, such as a math problem to be solved, or a crossword puzzle to be completed. But we can't compel our brains to produce only the thoughts we want and none of the thoughts we don't want. No one can.

The problem we have with worry isn't just that we don't control our thoughts. The problem is that we often forget that, or don't know it, and think that we *should* be controlling our thoughts. This leads us to an unnecessary and counterproductive wrestling match with our thoughts.

Why Do I Have These Thoughts?

Maybe you see the point I'm making about scary movies but still blame yourself for getting worried and afraid. Sometimes people point out to me that they could understand getting afraid while watching a scary movie, but they're getting afraid *without* the scary movie, and this is why they blame themselves.

It's true that they're not going to a theater in their external world, but they are watching a scary movie, of sorts. It's "in their head," in their internal world, in that space we all use for imagination. It's a private showing that's always open for an audience of one. It's a one-person show, a monologue of all kinds of unrealistic "what if" thoughts of unlikely calamities.

Why is this movie playing there, in your head? To understand this, you need to consider the purpose of anxiety.

What's the Purpose of Anxiety?

What do you think anxiety is good for? Why do we have the capacity to become anxious?

You're in the ballpark if you identified something about providing an alert to potential danger. It's to identify potential problems and threats, before they develop into a full blown crisis, so that we can devise solutions and live more safely. That's a good ability. We need that. More than any other species, probably, we have brains that give us the ability to imagine different future scenarios and plan responses. This is how some early hunter figured out how to trap huge mammoths in a pit where they could become food for the entire tribe. This ability helped us become the top predator on the planet, even in a world with bigger, stronger, and faster predators that had bigger teeth and claws.

A False Prediction

But this ability to imagine future developments isn't perfect. It can't be. We don't know the future until we get there, and our imagined projection of what will happen is subject to error. And there are only two possible types of errors.

Type One is called a "false positive." You believe something is present when it's not. If a caveman huddles in his cave all day, quaking with fear because he thinks he hears a saber-toothed tiger lurking nearby, when it's just a couple of rabbits that could be a meal for the clan, that's a false positive. He won't get eaten by a false positive, but it might prevent him from going outside and gathering food that he needs, or discovering that a nearby tribe is coming to attack him.

Type Two is called a "false negative." You believe something is absent when it's actually present. If a caveman strolls out of his cave, confident that there are no saber-toothed tigers around when one is quietly, patiently hiding behind some rocks, that's a false negative. The caveman can get eaten by a false negative.

No brain is error-free, so you have to have some kinds of errors. Which type would you choose? Thinking there's a tiger when there's none, or thinking there's no tiger when there is one? Our brains generally favor Type 1 errors over Type 2, and chronic worry is the result. This means you will probably never be surprised by a saber-toothed tiger, but you might instead spend a lot of time huddling in a dark, barren cave fearing tigers that aren't actually there, while daredevil tribes steal your crops and enjoy a meal of broiled rabbit.

Having a brain that favors Type 1 errors probably helped our species survive. And, like every other trait, it's distributed in different proportions among the population, just like height. Some people have a lot of this tendency, and some just a little. It helps the tribe to have some of both types of people— aggressive warriors who have so little fear that they will go out and bring home a mastodon for lunch, and cautious members who won't have any part of that, but will also live long enough to raise a new generation, and feed it by growing corn.

So there are advantages, at least to the species, to worrying. That's why we often have a tendency to worry. And some of us, by virtue of our genetic heritage, have more of a tendency than others. If you struggle with chronic worry, the odds are good that others who came before you in your family line had a similar struggle.

But, you might wonder, isn't this all learned? Haven't I trained myself to be a worrywart? And doesn't that make it my fault?

Is It All Your Fault?

No. You might be assuming that we're all born as a blank slate, that all our personalities and traits develop from learning, but it's not so. If you go to the maternity ward of your local hospital and see all the new babies, as the proud relatives come to see them there, you might notice how they all have different reactions to the lights and the noise. Some look directly at the source of noise and light and appear interested. Others cry and show signs of distress. Others show no interest either way. These are newborn babies, and yet they're clearly quite different from each other in their apprehension, and interpretation, of threat.

If you struggle with excessive chronic worry as an adult, there's a good chance this tendency goes back earlier in your life, even before it appeared to be a problem. You might stop to consider—did you show any tendencies toward extra worry in your childhood and early years? What stories do your parents and older siblings tell about you about this? It's frequently the case that this trait goes back a ways, even before people clearly recognized it for what it was.

Our brains didn't evolve to balance bank accounts, do quantum physics, or enjoy novels. They evolved to help us survive, by watching out for danger and solving problems. Brains that were more sensitive to danger—even if they saw ten tigers for every one that actually existed—had an advantage, and the people who had them were more likely to survive, and reproduce.

Our brains have the same basic function today—to watch for danger and solve problems. However, our environment has changed radically. We don't deal with saber-toothed tigers, rock slides, and swamps as much as we used to. Still, our brains continue to watch for bad possibilities, however remote and hypothetical, and try to figure out ways around them.

We also spend more time "in our heads" than our ancestors did. In modern civilizations, people spend much more time processing information—books, Internet, movies, and so on—than did our ancestors, who were much more focused on dealing with the physical objects in their environment. We get so used to working with thoughts that we often equate our thoughts with reality. We mistake the content that exists in our internal world for the objects and events that occur in our external world. It's not the same. That content is just our *thoughts* about the external world.

And, there's no off switch to the brain. It does this all the time, whether you like it or not. Like other vital functions that are important to our survival, it proceeds without our conscious control. That's why you see more scary movies in your head than you would otherwise choose, if it were entirely up to your conscious, deliberate choice.

Worry is not your enemy, although it can easily seem that way. If you have chronic worry, it can cause you a lot of trouble and unhappiness, and you will be much better off when you find a better way to relate to it. But chronic worry is not some terrible enemy that seeks to ruin your life. Nor is it some shameful flaw in your brain structure or your character. Chronic worry is more like a useful ability that has grown disproportionately large and influential even as the need for it has declined. Chronic worry is to ordinary worry as five pounds of chocolate is to one ounce. One will make you feel sick, while the other is a nice addition to your diet.

If you struggle with chronic worry, it's a problem, a problem to be solved or left unsolved. But don't get tricked into believing that it's your fault, or your enemy.

There's More to the Brain Than You Think

People often get very frustrated at their inability to talk themselves out of worrisome thoughts. "I know better than this," they'll say, "but it doesn't help!" They think the reason it doesn't help is that there's something wrong with them. However, the real reason is that a different part of the brain gets involved when you're afraid.

Most people, when they think about their brain, think about the part that's called the *cerebral cortex*. This is where conscious thought takes place, and it's where we use language and logic. There's a lot more to the brain, different parts that function differently. One of the other parts is called the *amygdala*. The amygdala has numerous functions, but one of its primary jobs is regulating the fear responses of fight and flight.

Meet Your Amygdala

I want to tell you a few things about the amygdala that will help you understand why you've been having so much trouble with chronic worry.

The amygdala handles fight and flight responses because it's capable of much faster action than the cerebral cortex. It has direct connections to our eyes and ears, getting information from the outside world before any other part of the brain. This rapid flow of information from the outside enables the amygdala to quickly answer the question, "Is it safe?"[1]

The amygdala doesn't use language. It learns by association, and that's how it remembers. So if you had a first panic attack in an Italian restaurant, you might thereafter have anxious thoughts and feel uneasy whenever you see a checkered tablecloth, or smell spaghetti sauce, and you might not know why. That's your amygdala at work, trying to keep you safe as it best knows how.

Your cerebral cortex can observe that there's no danger, just antipasto and garlic bread. At the movies, it can observe there's no monster, just a movie about monsters. Why doesn't the cerebral cortex tell the amygdala to stand down? Because the nervous connections between the amygdala and the cerebral cortex only allow for one-way communication. The amygdala can send signals to the cortex, but not the other way around.

This is a good thing because the amygdala is responsible for making rapid responses to dangerous circumstances. When a bus runs a red light and heads your way as you cross the street, your amygdala takes charge, and you find yourself darting out of the way without consciously identifying the problem and thinking of a solution. Whatever you happened to be thinking when the bus lurched in your direction is gone, because your cortex has been effectively silenced. You don't need thought with a runaway bus, you need quick action! We don't have time for all the conscious, deliberate thought of the cortex at that moment. Compared to the amygdala, the cortex is like a committee of old guys, sitting around reminiscing, arguing, and using more words than necessary to describe bus trips they've taken. It's too slow for emergencies!

This is why you can't calm down by telling yourself the worries are irrational. The amygdala isn't listening. It doesn't have time for all the yammering of your cerebral cortex. It's too busy watching for signs of trouble and responding, trying to protect you the only way it knows how—goading you into action by making you anxious.

Maybe you're thinking now that you'd like to tell your amygdala a thing or two. You can't! It doesn't use language! So how can you retrain your amygdala so it doesn't push the panic button when you're not really in danger?

Final fact you need about the amygdala: it only "learns," or creates new memories, when it's activated. Know what I mean by activated? I mean when you become afraid. When everything seems routine, and you're just going along with business as usual, your amygdala is on standby and not making any new memories. It's only when your amygdala detects what it takes as a sign of danger that it activates your sympathetic nervous system, enabling fight and flight responses, and then it will make memories.

Your opportunity to retrain your amygdala, and change your relationship with chronic worry, comes when you feel frightened or upset by your thoughts. If you had a dog phobia, you would retrain your amygdala by spending time with a dog, getting afraid, and hanging out with the dog long enough for the fear to subside. Then the amygdala would make some new observations about dogs, and as you repeatedly spent time with dogs, your chronic fear reaction would subside. You can't "tell" your amygdala that dogs are okay, but you can create the opportunities for it to discover that.

And if you're a person with chronic worry, the worrisome thoughts are your dogs. You can make progress the same way the person with a dog phobia makes progress—by working with your thoughts, rather than against them.

"Getting Through It" Misses the Point

When people get more fear than they bargained for in a scary movie, they often employ a variety of techniques to "get through it." They could leave the theater—some people do—but most want to stay if possible, usually because they came to the theater with a friend who wants to stay. So they do some things in an effort to hold the fear at bay while they remain in the theater.

Maybe they distract themselves by retying their shoelaces, or checking for text messages. Maybe they try some cognitive restructuring, reminding themselves "It's only a movie!" although they already knew that. Maybe they cover their ears or close their eyes, trying to take in less of the scary material. Maybe they grab onto the person next to them. (That works best if you came in with that person!)

The techniques people use to get through a scary movie resemble the techniques people often use with chronic worry. The safety behaviors you reviewed in chapter 3—involving efforts such as distraction, changing or correcting your thoughts, and reducing the cues or information coming to your attention—all work like these scary movie techniques. It's important to see that these techniques don't do much to relieve the worrying. Rather, they lock it in place, because they require constant repetition and monitoring, like plugging a leak with your finger. They establish an uneasy stalemate, like two equally matched people competing in a tug of war. And while these natural responses to the movie may help you stay in the theater, they probably won't help you become less afraid of the movie itself. If you were to see that movie again, you would probably have anticipatory thoughts about how scary it was and would be motivated to use the same avoidant techniques (closing eyes, distracting, and so on) you used the first time.

Since you probably don't plan to see it again, that's not a problem. However, when you use the same kind of techniques to respond to your worrisome thoughts, *this is a big problem.* While you probably won't see the movie again, you're going to reexperience those thoughts, again and again, because they're a naturally occurring part of life. If you handle your thoughts the same way you handle a one-time experience of a scary movie, you are locking in this unfortunate mental struggle, rather than relieving it. You're not changing how you relate to the worry. You're putting in more effort and struggle, which will maintain, rather than change, the unpleasant way you relate to the worry.

All Worry Means the Same Thing

We have a variety of ways of experiencing anxiety. For instance, we experience anxiety in the form of physical sensations. This might include such obvious symptoms as heart racing, muscular tension, labored breathing, stomach upset, sweating, trembling, and so on.

We also experience anxiety in the form of behaviors. Examples of behavioral anxiety would include some instances of nail biting, hair pulling, and other compulsive behaviors. Also included would be various forms of avoidance and escape—such as shopping for groceries at odd hours or in small stores, for fear of having to wait in a long line; driving on a local road rather than a highway even though it takes twice as long; taking a long trip by car rather than airplane, for fear of flying; eating lunch at your desk rather than the cafeteria because you experience social anxiety; and so on. Foot tapping, leg jiggling, fidgeting and shifting in one's seat, all kinds of restless movements of the body without apparent goal are also examples of behavioral expressions of anxiety.

We also experience anxiety in the form of thoughts.

These different types of symptoms all have the same essential meaning: *I'm nervous.* Over time, we come to learn what our nervous symptoms mean. The first few times people experience the sensations of a nervous stomach, they're likely to think those symptoms mean illness, maybe even vomiting. However, as they gain experience with these symptoms, people can come to recognize that the sensations are about being nervous, not ill.

The physical symptoms of a panic attack may fool a person over a longer period of time. It's not at all uncommon for people experiencing panic attacks to continue to believe, for an extended period, that the physical symptoms of a panic attack are warnings of death or loss of control. However, as people make progress with panic disorder, they come to recognize that the symptoms don't mean that at all. The symptoms simply mean they're feeling panicky.

How Your Thoughts Are Fooling You

Thoughts are trickier. With physical sensations and behaviors that are signs of anxiety, people naturally learn to interpret the symptoms accurately. If you see a person in a meeting, constantly jiggling his leg, how likely are you to think that this person really wants to play soccer, or to kick you? If you see someone biting a fingernail, how likely are you to think that this person is so hungry as to be reduced to eating fingernails? Probably not so likely! You would probably recognize that these symptoms have to be interpreted. It's overly simplistic to take the appearance of a symptom as its complete meaning.

But with thoughts (especially our own thoughts), it's easy to get fooled into taking the apparent content of the thought as the precise meaning of the thought. No interpretation appears necessary. If I experience a thought such as *What if I have cancer?* in an anxious frame of mind, I might very well respond as though the thought about cancer is itself a sign of cancer, when in fact the thought is simply an expression of nervousness which happens to be focused on the idea of cancer. In the same way, heart racing is a sign of nervousness that happens to be focused on the heart, and nail biting is a sign of nervousness that happens to be focused on the teeth and fingernails.

Ultimately, the real meaning of the worrisome thoughts of chronic worry generally has little to do with the apparent content and subject matter of the thoughts. We'll return to this topic in chapter 6, when we diagram the worry thoughts. The real meaning of these worrisome thoughts is the same as the meaning of the heart racing in someone experiencing a panic attack, the sweating and dry mouth experienced by someone preparing to give a presentation, or the jiggling of a leg as someone waits, idly, for a meeting to start or an airplane to take off.

What's that meaning? *I'm nervous.* Plain and simple—I'm nervous.

Yet, because these symptoms are expressed in words, or pictures, we tend to treat them differently than other symptoms. We have thoughts about thoughts. We have certain ideas about thoughts—what they mean, how we should respond to them—that often get in our way.

Finding a solution to the problem of chronic worry is going to involve new ways of responding to it, not efforts to abolish it.

Let's suppose that, instead of simply wanting to "get through" a scary movie, a movie that you previously found very upsetting, you wanted to get to a point where you could watch it without feeling any strong emotion. I don't know why you'd want that, but if that were your ambition, how could you get to the point where the movie didn't bother you so much?

The answer won't involve anything like those steps that people take to "get through" a scary movie. Those steps maintain the fear by struggling to keep it at bay. That's okay with a scary movie. It's okay to "get through" a scary movie because it's a very small, incidental part of your life, one you can leave behind when the show is over. However, worry can become a big part of life, and struggling to simply "get through" life itself is not a strategy, it's a tragedy.

The answer that occurs to me is that the most reliable way to drain a scary movie of the fear, to make it kind of tedious rather than fearsome, would be to watch that movie again and again. You could rent the DVD (or whatever technology is now current!) and view it over and over—not skipping the scary parts, not turning off the scary sound, but rather immersing yourself in it, again and again.

You'd need to have a strong motive to do this, because you'd feel unpleasantly afraid during the first several viewings. But do you have any doubt, if you watched it this way often enough, that it would gradually lose its ability to scare you?

After all, this is what naturally happens even to people who are fans of scary movies. A new scary movie will come out, and an aficionado will discover his new "favorite" scary movie. He'll go see that movie several times. And, after a number of viewings, he no longer derives as much scary "pleasure" as he used to, and sooner or later a new scary movie becomes his favorite. The old favorite becomes boring with repetition.

That's what we want to do with chronic worry, make it more boring and less upsetting.

How can you start doing that? The next two chapters will show you.

Thinking It Over

All too often, people take their chronic worry about unlikely events and exaggerated consequences to be a sign that there's something wrong with them. This leads them to blame and shame themselves, as if they had some terrible self-inflicted flaw, and to struggle against the worry in ways that maintain rather than remove it. I hope this chapter has helped you see how worry is a natural part of life, the side effect of an ability that has helped the human species survive and flourish, and that chronic worry is the result of trying to suppress that which can't—and needn't—be suppressed. The more you can cultivate an accepting attitude toward the thoughts of chronic worry, the easier your task will be.

What's a good way to do that? We'll take that up in the next chapter.

Putting Out Fires with Gasoline, and the Rule of Opposites

"The harder I try, the worse it gets."

If I had a nickel for every time a client said that to me, I'd need so many coin wrappers. Does this thought ever occur to you? Does it describe the history of your efforts to overcome chronic worry?

It's so frustrating! You work so hard to rid yourself of these unwanted, unhelpful worries, and get no lasting benefit from your effort. It often seems to make things worse, rather than better.

In fact, if you've been using methods like the ones described in chapter 3, you have been using methods which make things worse. You don't continue to have chronic worry *despite* your best efforts. You continue to have chronic worry *because* of your best efforts. It's the ultimate irony! Your efforts to stop worrying are the main reason you continue to worry.

Is It You, or Your Methods?

This might lead you to think there's something wrong with you, and to blame yourself for all the worrying. You might think that you'll always be burdened with this problem and feel different from all the "normal" people in your life who appear not to have any worries.

There's a valuable truth hidden behind the blame and shame. If you're trying to achieve something, and find that the harder you try the worse it gets, you should take a very close look at the methods you're trying. There's probably something about those methods that gives you the unwanted results. It's more likely the method that's defective, rather than you. You've gotten tricked into using methods that not only can't bring you the outcome you seek, but push it further away!

Chronic worry is one of those problems for which the metaphor "putting out fires with gasoline" was created. This metaphor describes a person who, on discovering a neighbor's house on fire, frantically grabs the nearest liquid he can find. Unfortunately, this turns out to be one of hundreds of buckets of gasoline in the yard. Even worse, in his haste he assumes the buckets contain water. He throws some gasoline on the fire, which burns even higher and hotter as a result. Seeing that the problem is growing, the man frantically throws even more gasoline, and the fire grows more, and so on. The harder he tries, the bigger the fire gets.

There are some problems with this metaphor—who doesn't recognize the smell of gasoline, and who keeps it in buckets around their home? But if we overlook these minor flaws, the story helps us evaluate the problem of chronic worry.

Suppose now that the neighbor, the one who collects gasoline for a hobby, returns home, and shouts, "Hey! This won't work! You're putting out fires with gasoline!"

What do you do? If you suddenly discover that you've been putting out fires with gasoline, you probably don't have any idea what to do next. You're upset with yourself for making this mistake, worried about how it will look to your neighbor whose house is burning, wishing that you had never gotten involved, and so on. On one hand, you don't know what to do. But on the other, the first step is really obvious.

Put down the buckets! Stop throwing that gasoline on the fire!

Almost anything will be better than throwing more gasoline on the fire. Standing there and doing nothing will be better! Don't try throwing the gasoline faster, or farther, or a little more to the left. Put down the gasoline!

What does this tell us about handling chronic worry? It suggests that, when we get caught up in chronic worry, our natural instinct of how to solve the problem turns out to be doing things that make the problem worse, rather than better. You probably have responses to worry—identified in the inventory you created in chapter 3—that you'll be better off without. Those are your buckets of gasoline.

Counterintuitive Problems

How could this happen? How can we go so far wrong as to make our situation worse by trying to make it better?

It's not hard, really, nor is it uncommon. Worry is a special kind of counterintuitive problem, one in which your gut instincts of how to help yourself are likely to make it worse rather than better. When you try to solve a counterintuitive problem with intuitive solutions, things usually get worse.

When my son, at two years old, would say "no" to everything, that was a counterintuitive problem for me. I would sometimes forget that he was learning to be independent, learning to use a powerful word, and that this was exciting and fun for him. Sometimes I would approach him as if I just needed to share my adult knowledge with him and help him see the error of his ways. So we would argue! The more we argued, the more he delighted in saying "no." His favorite phrase was "because not." (Now he's twenty, and we still do this occasionally, for old times' sake!)

If I try to solve a counterintuitive problem with an intuitive solution, I'm probably going to fail. If I want to solve a counterintuitive problem, I need a solution that is counterintuitive. I need to fight fire with fire.

This isn't as bizarre as it might sound. There are many everyday examples of this. I learned as a young child, when my puppy got off her leash, that if I chased her she would run away. She had four legs to my two, so the results were always poor. But if I ran away from her, she would chase me, and then I could grab her collar when she caught me. Counterintuitive.

When you're wading into the ocean, and a large wave comes toward you? If you turn and run for shore, the wave will probably break on your shoulders and knock you down. You'll swallow saltwater and sand. But if you dive into the base of the wave, it will pass right over you as if it were nothing. Counterintuitive.

Driving on an icy road, and starting to skid toward a phone pole? If you try to steer away from that pole, you'll probably be talking to your insurance agent soon. However, if you steer into the skid and aim for the pole (who was the brave guy that first figured this out?), you'll straighten out and be okay. Counterintuitive.

There are lots of counterintuitive problems. When the military trains soldiers to respond to an ambush, they train them to run toward the enemy, not away. Why? Well, the other side is expecting you to run away, and that's where they plan to shoot next (I hope they're not reading this!). If you're stuck in quicksand? Okay, you get the idea. Counterintuitive.

The difficulty with solving counterintuitive problems is that when you're trying so hard to solve a problem, and see that you're failing, your natural instinct is to "try harder," and that makes things worse. It can almost feel like an insult when the world doesn't respond to your solution. This often leads people to get frustrated and upset with themselves while they continue to make things worse.

Attitudes about Thoughts

The previous examples all involve counterintuitive problems in the world around us. It's even trickier when we have counterintuitive challenges in our internal world, in our own minds. We have some unexamined assumptions about our thoughts that influence our reactions in unhelpful ways.

Our brains are not like computers that simply generate output. A computer generates an answer to a problem—maybe it calculates something for you, or maybe it formats material you've written into a letter format—and it has no opinion about what it produced. You "ask" a computer a question, and that's all you get, the answer.

Not so with our brains. We have thoughts, including worries. We also have attitudes, beliefs, and thoughts *about* our thoughts. One belief about thoughts that we briefly examined in chapter 3 is the belief that thoughts can be dangerous. Let's take another look at that.

Are Thoughts Dangerous? Want to try an experiment? Take a minute now to think about this book catching fire in your hands. Think about it in great detail. Picture the flames curling the pages, the white pages turning to gray ash, the smell of burnt paper, the smoke spiraling toward the ceiling. Any minute the smoke alarm should start screeching a warning. And yet here you are, still holding the unburned book in your hands, reading these words.

It seems clear that thoughts aren't dangerous. Only actions can be dangerous.

Why Can't You Just Control Your Thoughts?

One important attitude that many people hold about their thoughts is that they "ought" to be in control of them. They think they should be able to have the thoughts they want and not have the thoughts they don't want. Do you think about it this way?

People who hold this belief are often offended and irritated by the way their thoughts seem to defy them. Again and again, they review the evidence about the content of their worries and see that the feared events are not at all likely to occur. They tell themselves that there's "nothing to worry about." Then they go on about their business. Sooner or later, they find themselves having the same worrisome thoughts. Maybe they've even been watching for them! Then they get mad at themselves all over again, wondering "why" they keep having the same dumb thoughts, reprimanding themselves the same way you might reprimand a teenager who has once again left dirty dishes on the table instead of clearing them away.

The truth is, we don't have pinpoint control of our thoughts. And there's *always* something to worry about, because we can worry about any possibility we can imagine. We don't need realistic danger to worry.

Try This Experiment. Think of an elephant for about twenty seconds, and then stop thinking of it. No more elephant. Take one minute and keep it out of mind. No long trunk, no loud trumpeting sound, no tusks, no eating peanuts, no running away from mice.

How did you do? Odds are you just spent some time with thoughts of elephants. For most people, the results will be as obvious as an elephant stomping through the jungle. And if it seems to you as though you had no thoughts of elephants during that minute, then ask yourself this question: how do you know? The only way you can try to avoid all thoughts of elephants is to think of what it is to think about elephants, and watch to see if you do that while trying not to do it! You get elephants on the brain from every direction!

Anytime you deliberately try to stop thinking of something, you're likely to think more about it. Psychological research on the subject of thought suppression[1] clearly shows that the main effect of thought suppression is a resurgence of the thoughts you're trying to forget.

It's the same with our emotions. We don't control our thoughts or our emotions—or our physical sensations, for that matter. The more we try, the more we get thoughts and feelings we don't want.

Your lack of direct control over thoughts and emotions may come to your attention quite clearly when some well-meaning friend tries to help you by saying "Don't think about it" or "Calm down!" It's probably painfully obvious to you what's wrong with that suggestion. It might even make you angry that this person "doesn't get it." And yet, you may be continually trying to use this strategy without noticing that you're using the same unhelpful method that doesn't work, and then getting disappointed and frustrated when it fails again. If it doesn't work when a friend urges you to "calm down," it's probably not going to work when you urge it upon yourself!

What Do We Really Control?

People often assume that control is measured by what they think and feel. They think that if they're having odd or illogical thoughts, or strongly unpleasant and exaggerated emotions, that this means they're "out of control." They don't like that idea, so they struggle to control their thoughts and feelings, and this is like trying to grab a greased pig on ice. The more you try to control thoughts and feelings, the more out of control they seem.

Control is about *what we do*, not what we think and feel. That's why our laws describe behavior that's expected and restricted. Society expects people to control what they do—how they drive, how they treat others, how they wait their turn in line, and so on. Our laws and social norms aren't based on what people think and feel because nobody really controls those things. Control is about what you do.

And yet, it's part of the human condition to assume that we can, or should be able to, control our thoughts and emotions. Certainly there are times when we want to. Our intuitive instinct with respect to worry is to "stop thinking that." And it backfires, because worry is a counterintuitive problem. You'll be better off with a counterintuitive solution for this counterintuitive problem.

Thinking: It's Just What the Brain Does

Your brain is an organ and, like other organs—stomach, kidneys, liver—it has tasks to accomplish. Your stomach digests food. Your kidneys remove waste products from the bloodstream and produce urine. And your brain, among other things, identifies problems and generates solutions. Actually, most of the work our brains do (maintaining balance, monitoring the work of other organs and glands, watching for emergencies, and so on) takes place without our awareness. The brain activity that gets our attention—the thinking, calculating, verbal work—is actually a very small portion of the brain's activity, taking place in the cerebral cortex.

An ancient proverb tells us, "The mind is a wonderful servant, but a terrible master." The brain is a useful tool. We can direct our attention and thoughts to topics in order to design bridges, land a rocket on an asteroid, and calculate our taxes. Left without enough to do, however, the brain is likely to cause mischief as it generates thoughts on its own.

If you go too long without eating, your stomach will start to do digestive things without any food to digest, and you will feel abdominal discomfort, hear your stomach make embarrassing noises, and so on. It's trying to fulfill its purpose even when it doesn't have the necessary ingredients. It's the same with your brain. If your brain doesn't have enough problems to solve, it will make some up and try to solve them.

That's chronic worry—your brain making up problems and trying to solve them, and you taking those thoughts as seriously as you take the tax calculations.

You've probably noticed that you experience more worry when you're not so busy, and that when you're really busy with activities and problems to solve you don't seem to worry nearly as much. Maybe you've tried to use "keeping busy" as a way to cut back on your worrying. This is why. Worry is a leisure time activity. It expands, or contracts, to fill the time that's available, because it's simply not as important as most of our other activities. It takes what's left over. Your brain is literally acting like a bored puppy, chewing on the carpet because it doesn't have enough things to do.

We can train that puppy well enough that it will no longer chew on furniture, especially if we offer him other things to chew on. However, we can't train the brain not to think of problems (because that's a main purpose of the brain), any more than we could train our stomach not to rumble when we're hungry.

Instead, we need to change the way we relate to our worry. We do better by learning how to accept and work with, rather than oppose, that fact that we are experiencing worry thoughts. We will also do better when we can recognize the worry thoughts as signs of nervousness and anxiety, the same as an eye twitch or sweaty palms, rather than some important message about the future.

Rules of Life

I regularly teach workshops for professional therapists about the treatment of anxiety disorders, and I usually like to introduce the workshop with an expanded and embellished version of the polygraph metaphor, commonly used in acceptance and commitment therapy.[2] Before I say hello, or introduce myself, before I say anything at all, I tell them this story.

> So a man walks into my office, someone I know as a man of his word, who says what he means and does what he says. This man walks into my office and he has a gun, and he says, "Now Dave, what I'd like for you to do is take all the furniture here in your office, and move it out into the waiting room…or else I'm gonna shoot you!"

"So," (*I ask the audience, and now I'll ask you, the reader*), "as students of human behavior, what is the outcome you predict here?"

And someone in the audience will say, "You're gonna move the furniture!"

That's right, I move the furniture—I can do that—I move the furniture and I live.

A week goes by and the man returns—same man, same gun—and he says "Now Dave, the thing I'd like for you to do, is sing the 'Star Spangled Banner.' The first verse will be sufficient. Sing the 'Star Spangled Banner,' or else I'm gonna shoot you."

So, what's the outcome you predict here?

I sing the song—I can do that—and I live.

Another week goes by, and once again the man appears, and this time he has a colleague with him. The colleague rolls a cart, full of electronic equipment, into my office. The man says, "Now Dave, my associate here, he's got lie-detecting equipment. The best electronics on the planet for detecting human emotion, virtually infallible. I'm gonna ask my associate to hook you up to the lie-detecting equipment. Then I just want you to relax. Or else I'm gonna shoot you."

What's the outcome you predict here?

Nothing good! Nothing good will come out of this one!

That allows me to get to the point of the story, namely, that this is the circumstance of some 40 million Americans with a chronic anxiety disorder. They wake up day after day, worried about feeling anxious, trying so hard not to feel anxious, and getting more anxious as a result of all that effort, digging a deeper hole with all their efforts to resist the anxiety. To help people overcome an anxiety disorder, therapists have to help people discover this aspect of the problem and learn to handle it differently.

And if you struggle with chronic worry, the same applies to your efforts to overcome that problem.

What makes it so apparent that I can move the furniture to save my life, and I can sing a song to save my life, but I can't relax to save my life?

From the perspective of acceptance and commitment therapy (ACT), the answer lies with two important rules of thumb that govern our lives.³ ACT is a form of therapy that, more or less, belongs within the school of cognitive behavioral therapy, but has some very different ideas from traditional CBT, particularly with respect to our efforts to control thoughts, emotions, and physical sensations.

First, there's a rule of thumb which governs our interactions with the external world around us, the physical environment that we live in. In the external world, the rule of thumb is something like this: the harder you try, and the more you struggle, the more likely you are to get what you want. Nothing is guaranteed, but you can improve your odds at getting something you want by making every effort possible. That's the rule of thumb that governs our interactions with the external world.

But that's not the only rule we live by. There's a second rule of thumb, one that pertains to our internal world of thoughts, emotions, and physical sensations. In this world, the rule is quite different. Here the rule is something like this: the more you oppose your thoughts, emotions, and physical sensations, the more you will have of them.

The rule that governs your internal world of thoughts, emotions, and physical sensations is the opposite of the rule that governs the external world. God help you if you didn't get the memo about the second rule, and you try to manage your thoughts, emotions, and physical sensations the same way you handle the world around you. It will lead you to use solutions that are bound to fail, and bring you grief and frustration every time.

If you're someone who struggles with chronic worry, only to find that the peace and calm you seek continues to elude you, then you're probably someone who will benefit by making more use of the second rule.

Our gut instinct, however, is usually to treat everything the same—oppose what we don't want, wherever it is. Let's now consider a workaround for this instinct: the Rule of Opposites.

The Rule of Opposites

This is an important rule of thumb which applies to a lot of anxiety symptoms. When we apply it to chronic worry, it means this:

My gut instinct of how to respond to unwanted, chronic worry is pretty much dead wrong. I am usually better off doing the opposite of my gut instinct.

How can this possibly be? Let's recall the worry trick from chapter 1: You experience doubt, and treat it like danger.

The worry trick is a powerful influence. It will be very helpful for you to understand what gives it such power.

How Can We Protect Against Danger?

What's good for danger? Three things: fight, flight, and freeze. If it looks weaker than me, I'll fight it. If it looks stronger than me, but slower, I'll run away from it. And if it looks stronger and faster than me, I'll freeze and hope it doesn't see so well. That's all we have for danger.

Fight/flight/freeze methods all involve opposing the worry—struggling to stop worrying; getting mad at yourself because you worry; fighting to distract yourself or to stop thinking of it; repeatedly seeking reassurance, from friends and the Internet, in an effort to stop worrying; thought stopping; reliance on drugs and alcohol; superstitious rituals; and all other manner of "fighting to calm down."

Doubt, however, isn't danger. It's just discomfort. And what's good for discomfort? A million variations on "chill out and let it pass." Claire Weekes, an Australian physician whose books about anxiety are still useful and popular fifty years later, recommended that people "float" through their anxiety.[4] People were often unclear about what she meant by float. I think she meant, literally, the opposite of swim. Make no effort. Simply allow the environment to support you, and go on with your business.

For danger, we fight, or run, or freeze. For discomfort, we chill out and give it time to pass. What's good for danger is the opposite of what's good for discomfort. So if you get tricked into treating worry as a danger, this naturally makes it worse.

When you treat worry as a danger that must be stopped or avoided, you're fighting fire with gasoline. Your gut instinct is actually pretty much the opposite of what would help. This is what gives the worry trick its power.

It's as if your compass is off by 180 degrees, showing north when it points south. If you have a compass that's off by 180 degrees, you can still find your way home, as long as you remember that the compass points the wrong way, and you need to go in the opposite direction it suggests.

Your gut instinct of how to handle worry has probably been to take its content seriously, opposing it and seeking to avoid it. That's what we saw in chapter 3. When you take worry to be a sign of danger, you naturally treat it that way.

We need something very different for the discomfort and doubt of worry. This way would allow us to recognize the doubts and uncertainties that occur to us, and also allow for the way our brains may be over-vigilant in imagining future dangers. It would allow us to distinguish between thoughts that occur in our brains (our internal world) and events that occur (or don't) in the external world. It would allow us to live more comfortably with the reality that we don't control our thoughts, and that our thoughts are not always our best guide to what is happening, or will be happening, in our external world.

The Rule of Opposites can be a powerful guide in the search for a more adaptive way to respond to worry. We'll come back to it again as we look for different methods you can use in responding to worry.

Thinking It Over

In this chapter, we reviewed the nature of worry and found it to be a counterintuitive problem, one best served by a counterintuitive response. This aspect of worry is firmly embedded in the Rule of Opposites, which suggests that a person's gut instinct of how to handle worry is usually wrong, dead wrong, and that we're better off doing the opposite of that instinct when it comes to handling worry. This rule will be an important guide as we consider different ways to work with worry.

The Mad Libs of Anxiety: Catch the Worries Before They Catch You

If you experience chronic worry and struggle to get a handle on it, here's one aspect of it you can turn to your advantage. Almost all of your worries—and I really mean all, like 99.9 percent of your worries—will announce themselves when they enter your mind. It's as if the worry were waving a big flag, to make sure you know it's arrived. Chronic worries almost always start with two particular words, the most overworked words in the vocabulary of a worrier.

You probably know this. What are the two words?

Think back to the last couple of times you struggled with a worrisome thought. What were the first few words of that thought?

What Are a Worrier's Two Most Over-Used Words?

You nailed it if you answered "What if…?"

Now I say this is an advantage, because these two words can point out to you that you're being lured into worry as surely as the sound of a starter pistol indicates the start of a race, or the siren of an ambulance behind you indicates the need to pull over.

Maybe you don't think that's an advantage! You might be so accustomed to trying to suppress and ignore your worrisome thoughts that anything that brings attention to them seems unhelpful. It might seem to you that you've been barely holding back the tide of unwanted worry, and that you'd be better off keeping it out of your awareness.

And yet, we saw in chapter 3 that "anti-worry" techniques usually make the problem of chronic worry more chronic and severe. Such techniques look like helpful solutions, but they're actually wolves in sheepdog's clothing. So bear with me! Suspend any disbelief on this point, at least until you've digested this chapter.

The "what if" words are a useful signal. However, if you're like most chronic worriers, you probably don't often notice them, and you may well underestimate how often this phrase appears in your thoughts and conversation.

"What if" probably sneaks around your attention the same way a pickpocket does. You're more likely to notice, and react to, the phrase that comes *after* the "what if…?" That's where all the upset of chronic worry comes from. "What if" is the bait that gets you to bite into something that will give you a real bellyache.

You can't change your relationship with worry if it catches you unawares. So it will probably be real helpful for you to get better at noticing the "what if" words and taking in their meaning. That will set the stage for you to start training yourself to respond differently to the worry, and developing a new way of relating to it. If this sounds like the opposite of what you've been trying—well, this is why we have the Rule of Opposites!

Let's start this work by diagramming the typical worry sentence. It's no longer part of the standard grade school curriculum, but when I attended grade school, we learned grammar by diagramming sentences. We'll do something similar here.

Diagram the Worry Sentence

Here's the actual structure of the overwhelming majority of chronic worries. It's composed of two clauses.

What if... _____?

(Insert catastrophe here)

It starts with the "what if?" clause. It's followed by the *catastrophe clause.*

Let's consider the "what if" clause for a moment. What does the "what if" clause mean here? What are we trying to convey when we say "what if"? What meaning does it add to the sentence?

You might not be so sure of what I'm getting at here, so let me explain. Think about when we're likely to get into "what if" thinking. If a dog comes up and bites me, how likely am I to say, or think, "What if a dog bites me?" Not very likely, right? I'm just gonna say, "Ouch!"

If a dog comes up to me and growls, fur on end, showing teeth, and in every way looking like a dog about to attack, how likely am I to be thinking, *What if this dog bites me?* Still not very likely, right? I'm much more likely to be looking around for the dog's owner, or a stick I can use to defend myself, a fence I can hop, or a tree I can climb. I'm going to be focused on protecting myself any way I can.

So when do I say (or think), "What if a dog bites me?" What do you think?

I think the answer is: when I'm neither being bitten nor about to be bitten. I don't say it when a dog has his teeth on my leg. I don't say it when a dog is in front of me, preparing to attack. I'm too busy protecting myself to be thinking much of anything! I say, or think, "What if a dog bites me?" when I'm *not* being threatened by a dog; I say it, or think it, when my cerebral cortex has center stage, and my amygdala is on standby in the background. For instance, if I had a dog phobia, I might have this thought just as I was ready to leave the house, ready to walk a few blocks to catch my train. However, if a dog actually charges me while I'm walking to the train, my amygdala will take charge, silence the blabbing of my cortex, and fill me with the energy and the urgency I need to protect myself. That conversation with the committee of old guys will have to wait until I'm no longer threatened by the dog!

Dog attacks don't cause worrying—they cause self-protection!

So what meaning does the "what if" clause add to our sentence?

It means "let's pretend."

Does that work for you? Does that describe the meaning of "what if" that appears in your worries? "Here's something that's not happening in the external world now, and let's pretend it is."

It's actually more specific than that. When's the last time you found yourself thinking, *What if I wake up tomorrow, feeling real good, happy with myself and my place in the world, love in my heart for everyone, knowing that those feelings will last for the rest of my life?*

Not so recently, right? In fact, probably never! People generally don't "what if" about good stuff. It's all about negative, terrible, dreadful things that could possibly happen in the future.

So "what if" really means "Let's pretend something bad."

Maybe, though, you're thinking it really means "This could happen," or "It's possible that..." You might think that this could be an important signal about some bad thing that is possible. If this is the case, I have another question for you.

What would be some things that are clearly, irrefutably impossible?

Take your time, but I don't think you'll come up with much. There's really nothing that seems impossible if we think about it long enough. That's one of the differences between your internal world and the external world. In the external world, there are rules that govern reality. In our minds, there are no rules. We can imagine anything, no matter how improbable or impossible, and be unable to *prove* that it's impossible.

This doesn't give you much guidance to live by. And our "what if" thoughts don't cover all the things that seem possible—just the really bad ones. This is how my wife and I ended up so concerned with my son's jaundice, as I explained in chapter 1.

What goes in the catastrophe clause? Whatever you happen to be most worried about that day, week, month, or year. It's a fill-in-the-blank choice, and if you're presently most worried about your job, or your health, or your spouse, or your furnace, that's what's going to show up there.

So here's what we have:

Let's pretend... _____.

(Some catastrophe)

The "what if" part of chronic worry is all about pretending. When chronic worry tricks you into pretending something is true, it doesn't matter how important or unimportant that pretend content is. Pretending is like multiplying by zero! It doesn't matter how big a number is, when you multiply by zero, you still end up with nothing.

Worrying About "What If?" Is Like a Game

Do you know the game Mad Libs? It's a party game that became real popular in the 1960s. It was a book full of very short stories that had words missing. You'd get a bunch of your friends together and then you'd ask them to give you the words you needed to complete the story, without letting them see the story. You'd tell them "give me an adverb—a color—a number—a proper noun," and so on. You'd write these words in where they were needed, and then you'd read the completed story to your friends. Then they'd laugh, especially if you had served plenty of beer beforehand. This is what we did for fun before the Internet.

So, this "what if" sentence, this statement of chronic worry, this is the Mad Libs of anxiety. It's just as arbitrary, as random, as that. You can fill in a catastrophe here, any catastrophe. It doesn't matter what you pick. You have your usual choices— your "favorite" worries—but they all fit! They all fit because you have "Let's pretend" in front.

The problem is, after a while you forget that you're pretending.

If you're like most people with chronic worry, over time you get so used to these thoughts that you stop noticing the pretend part. You probably don't even notice the "what if" clause after a while. The only part of the thought you consciously notice is the inflammatory and exaggerated catastrophe clause.

When you don't notice the "what if" clause, you get this steady drumbeat of ideas in your mind that suggest disaster. You don't notice the part that tells you it's pretend! No wonder people can get so anxious and depressed in response to worry. It's like a cable TV channel devoted exclusively to bad news, beamed directly into your mind.

When you don't notice the "what if" clause, this drumbeat of ideas sounds like this:

What if...I GET CANCER?

What if...MY SPOUSE LEAVES ME?

What if... I FREAK OUT DURING MY PRESENTATION?

What if...I GET SO NERVOUS, THEY THINK I'M A TERRORIST?

What if...I LOSE MY MIND AT THE RESTAURANT OVER LUNCH?

The effect of the worry is strengthened even more by the fact that it often occurs while you're multitasking. Even if you noticed the "what if" part, you don't have the opportunity to give it your full attention and resolve it. You're too busy checking your text messages while eating your lunch and scanning your schedule. This thought has a lot of subliminal power. We don't stop to notice that we're experiencing this particular thought and respond to the thought as just that, a thought. Instead, we skip right past the "what if" part, focus in on the catastrophe clause, and absorb its message as if it were true.

This is one of the obstacles you face in dealing with the problem of worry. As a society, we value thought, and usually think of thought as one of our characteristics that sets us apart from animals, one of the highlights of billions of years of evolution. We value human thought. And most of us are vain enough to put a particularly high value on our own thought. Thought is good, powerful, and important, we believe, and *my thoughts* are especially good, powerful, and important. We certainly act this way in responding to worry. If we didn't take these thoughts to be important, they wouldn't cause us so much grief!

Our brains are wonderful problem-solving tools. More than any other factor (except perhaps opposable thumbs), it's our brains that have enabled us to become the top predator of the planet. Our brains have produced the wheel, speech and writing, and the calculations necessary to land a ship on a comet.

But the brain is still a problem-solving organ, looking for problems to solve. And, especially when there's no urgent problem (like an attacking dog) to solve, the brain will make up some problems, just to have something to do. So it doesn't matter how smart you are. A certain amount of your thoughts will just be noisy nonsense.

How Worry Baits You

This "what if" clause is like that red flag to a bull that I mentioned in chapter 4. Imagine if you could have a heart-to-heart conversation with a bull, just before a bullfight. I think it would go something like this.

> Listen, bull, I know how you feel when you see that red flag. Your blood boils, right? You want to paw the ground, snort real loud, then race over and flatten that flag, and the guy holding it, too. But remember what happened to your cousin, Toro? He ran over to that flag, and while he was attacking it, some guys stuck

short knives in his side. Then another guy waved it again, and when Toro ran at him, the guy stabbed him in the neck with a sword. It was a trick! They bait you with that red flag, man! So the best thing for you to do, when they start waving that thing at you, is remember it's a trick! Lie down and eat some daisies! Don't take the bait! Don't get suckered!

It would be real hard to train a bull to do that. But you can train yourself to take a pass on the "what if" bait, to notice the "what if" and respond differently. You can train yourself to remember that it is, in fact, a bunch of bull.

The first step is to get better at consciously noticing the "what if" clause. This is the part that says "Let's pretend (something bad)," and when you don't notice this clause, it's easy to lose sight of the pretending. Generally, the catastrophe clause that follows seems so upsetting and ominous that it's easy to forget about the "what if" part, especially when you barely noticed it to begin with.

So here's a way to become more aware of the "what if" clause.

Count Your Worries

Get yourself some bottles of Tic Tacs, or any kind of mint that comes in fixed quantities. Tic Tacs, for instance, come in bottles of sixty and one hundred (except in Australia, where they come in bottles of fifty—go figure!), but any kind of mint or candy that comes in a fixed number per bottle will do. Keep it with you at all times, in your pocket, purse, or briefcase.

Get into this habit. Whenever you notice a "what if" thought (or you hear yourself saying it out loud), take out your bottle of Tic Tacs. Take one out. You can eat it, or you can flick it onto the street, or toss it in the garbage. Whatever you do with it is fine, just remove one from the bottle and close the bottle.

You can use this as a way to track, and count, the number of times you experience a *What if...?* thought during the week. If you prefer, you could use some other method, like a clicker. I like the Tic Tacs, though, because they are more likely to interrupt you in your mental "business as usual." And, if you feel self-conscious about doing this kind of self-monitoring, no one will notice a thing—just a person eating a mint!

Practice makes permanent. Do this for a couple of weeks, and you will make a pretty permanent change in your ability to notice the "what if" thoughts. They will no longer be subliminal, slipping into your mind unnoticed the way a pickpocket gets your wallet without drawing your attention. Now you will become more and more aware of the habit. And it will start to lose some of its power to fool you.

Most people quickly come to recognize how central these "what if" words are. Occasionally I meet someone who discovers they use a variation on this phrase, such as "Suppose," "Isn't it possible," or other words that contain the same invitation to imagine bad stuff happening in the future. If you discover that your worry bait comes in a slightly different wording, you can use Tic Tacs to observe that wording as well.

One more thing before you start. As you start using the Tic Tacs, you might be displeased when you notice how many times you catch yourself in the act of "what if"-ing. You might feel overwhelmed when you realize how often this thought occurs to you. You might feel, initially, that you would have much preferred that I hadn't ever brought it to your attention.

Don't be fooled. This is the good news, when you notice all those "what if"s, even though you may initially feel dismayed and discouraged. It's the good news because you've been having all those thoughts for some time, long before you started this book. All that's different now is that you're noticing them. That's the good news, because noticing them is a new skill that will help you.

Keep track of your counts for a couple of weeks to help you really get into this habit of passively observing "what if."

How does this strategy of becoming more consciously aware of these "what if" thoughts compare to what you usually do?

I'm thinking that it's probably the *opposite* of what you usually do. That might seem odd and uncomfortable to you. However, it's actually a good sign that your efforts to change your relationship with chronic worry are on the right track.

Remember the Rule of Opposites: "My gut instinct of how to respond to chronic worry is typically dead wrong, and I am better off doing the opposite of my gut instinct." (If you don't remember that, you can review it in chapter 5.)

If you keep responding in the same way, you can expect the same results. We're looking for different results here, and this will take different, even opposite, actions.

We can see the Rule of Opposites in action when we consider that many people try very hard to distract themselves from their worrisome thoughts. If that really worked, you wouldn't be reading this book. You would have already dismissed and banished your unwanted worries.

It just doesn't work that way. It works the opposite. The more you try to eject thoughts from your mind, the more they keep coming back in, like unwanted drunks at a party.

That doesn't mean the effort to distract yourself is worthless, however. It can point to some useful information. Consider this question: When you are motivated to distract yourself from a problem, what does it tell you about that problem?

Think about that for a minute. What kind of problems do we usually want to distract ourselves from?

Imagine that you were standing in line at a bank when a robbery broke out, and you heard gunshots. How likely would you be to take out your checkbook and balance it, in order to distract yourself from the unpleasant gunplay?

Probably not very likely! You'd be too busy diving to the floor, or looking for some cover or an exit. You'd be trying to protect yourself, not distract yourself.

When are we motivated to distract ourselves from unpleasant and worrisome thoughts? When we're not facing a clear and present danger. When the chips are not down. When the babbling of our cerebral cortex, rather than the self-defense of our amygdala, is center stage.

So when you notice that you feel the urge to distract yourself, this can be a powerful reminder of what the game is. The chips are not down, you are not in danger, and that's why you are motivated to distract. If you actually *were* under the gun, you wouldn't even think of distraction!

The "Why?" Question

The "what if?" question is the pickpocket that steals your peace of mind, and it does it so sneakily that you don't notice what's actually happening.

Most pickpockets have an accomplice, someone who draws the attention of potential victims away from the pickpocket by clumsily bumping into people, or even shouting out "Watch out for pickpockets!" on a crowded train. When people get bumped, or hear a warning about pickpockets, they tend to check their wallets, which tells the pickpocket where they are. Pickpockets understand the Rule of Opposites.

The "why?" question is the pickpocket's accomplice.

When you're having the thought that you should be controlling your brain and find that once again, your brain is producing all kinds of unreasonable and unwanted worrisome thoughts, you're likely to respond with "why" questions, such as "*Why* do I keep worrying so much?"

People usually experience the "why" question as a kind of rhetorical question. They don't really expect an answer. It's more of a protest, a finger-pointing question, an angry demand that some higher authority correct this injustice. It's not a question so much as a complaint. Unfortunately, it's a complaint expressed in the absence of a complaint department. This question leads people to feel weaker and more pessimistic about their future, because it suggests that the solution to the problem requires someone else, maybe even God, to do something. Meanwhile, they have to wait and worry.

When you're caught up in worry, getting into the "why" question amounts to taking the bait. The "why" question is usually some form of resistance to the worry, rather than an actual inquiry. And resistance to worry inevitably fans the flames of worry, rather than extinguishing them. This resistance is the equivalent of slamming on the brakes when my car starts skidding on an icy road. That's the last thing I need! Resistance is intuitive. It's also counterproductive. What we really need is a response that's counterintuitive and productive.

People often think that the "why" question is the key issue. Why do I have these thoughts? Why me? Why here? Why now?

Better Questions

The truth is, "why?" is the least useful question there is about worry. This question is just another way of being anxious. While you probably can't simply dismiss it and make it go away, you don't have to get involved in taking it seriously. It will be more helpful to steer away from this "why" question, to catch yourself in the act of asking it, to notice it and move on to the more useful questions of "what and how."

What am I experiencing now? Well, I'm experiencing worrisome thoughts.

How can I respond to it? I'll cover this with the steps in chapter 9.

Thinking It Over

This chapter directed your attention to two types of worrisome thoughts—*What if...?* and *Why?*—that consistently mislead and misdirect you into a life of chronic worry, and suggested ways of disarming them. Becoming more aware of these thoughts as they occur to you is a big step in learning how to disregard the "bait" that so often lures people into making their worry more persistent.

CHAPTER 7

Thinking About Thoughts

It's a tricky thing to think about worry, because worry is thought. Things get complicated when we think about our thoughts, let alone try to change those thoughts. This chapter will take a look at the difficulties that can arise when people set out to change their thoughts, and ways around some of these difficulties.

Cognitive Behavioral Therapy for Anxiety

The introduction of cognitive behavioral therapy in the mid-1980s was a major breakthrough for people who suffered with chronic anxiety. Prior to this, there were very few good options for people who suffered with chronic anxiety. Now, for the first time, a method was introduced that offered practical, concrete ways to reduce chronic anxiety.

CBT was a radical departure from previous schools of therapy, and combined a cognitive (thinking) approach with a behavioral approach. On the cognitive side, it said that mistaken and exaggerated thoughts were heavily involved in producing and maintaining anxiety, and it offered a way to help clients identify and change those thoughts. The primary tool it

offered was cognitive restructuring, which involved the identi-
fication of various "errors of thinking" and the subsequent
review and correction of these thoughts.

Identifying Worrisome Thoughts

So, for instance, a person who struggled with lots of worry
about money and job security would be directed to identify his
key worrisome thoughts on the subject. These thoughts might
include statements like the following:

I'm likely to get fired.

If I lose this job, I'm ruined.

I'm too old to get another job.

I'll never be able to support myself and my family again.

My wife will leave me, and I'll have to live in my car.

Since emotions are believed to be shaped by our thoughts
and beliefs about the topic, his emotions would be shaped by
these thoughts regardless of how true or false they were. If this
man's thoughts about finances and employment were exaggerated or unrealistic in some way, he would have an emotional
response in his internal world which was out of proportion to
his actual circumstances in the external world.

A CBT therapist would ask him to evaluate his thoughts
on the topic he worried about to see how realistic or unrealistic
they were, and to look for some characteristic errors in his
thoughts, as described in chapter 3. If this man found errors in
his typical thinking about employment and finances, he would
work to correct his thoughts, replacing the unrealistic thoughts
with more realistic versions. If these new, and more accurate,

thoughts about his situation were less negative and foreboding than his previous thoughts, this would change his emotional response for the better.

Changing Behavior

On the behavioral side, CBT would suggest changes in one's behavior that would ultimately reduce anxiety. This would include practicing with the objects, locations, and activities that people fear. So snake phobics would make progress by spending time with a snake, rather than avoiding it, and the same would apply to people who feared heights, shopping malls, driving, flying, and so on. Relaxation and meditative methods might also be used to lower overall anxiety levels, but exposure to what one fears is considered to be the most effective behavioral method by far.

Traditional CBT methods have been of enormous help to millions who had been suffering from chronic anxiety and worry. However, there are a few difficulties when we attempt to apply these methods to chronic worry.

For one, typical worry thoughts usually express uncertainty about a possibility, and most often begin with "what if" as in *What if I lose my job?* This type of worry isn't a prediction that can be evaluated and shown to be true or false. It's an invitation, as I point out in chapter 6, to "pretend" that something bad will happen and to worry about it. Since most hypothetical events, however likely or unlikely, are possible rather than impossible, this makes it more difficult to apply the usual tools of cognitive restructuring.

No matter how much evidence you may muster to show that you're unlikely to lose your job, chronic worry can always trump that argument by responding, "But what if you do?" This usually leads people to try to become "sure" that the feared event won't happen. When they can't do that, it serves to prolong and maintain the worry.

Secondly, the invitation to use cognitive restructuring to correct "errors of thinking" can mislead people into believing or hoping that we can tame, maybe even perfect our thoughts. This contains the implicit suggestion that we can do such a good job of correcting our thoughts as to eliminate dysfunctional worry.

This is a bridge too far, in my view, a hope that is more misleading than helpful. In my professional work as a psychologist, I have seen far too many people who struggled to correct their thoughts, who tried so hard to stop having unrealistic worries and thoughts which daily filled them with discomfort and upset, only to feel like failures because they failed to control their thoughts.

Your Brain Is Not a Computer

People often mistakenly think of their brain as a computer. Let's suppose you're running a program which doesn't work exactly the way you want. Maybe it has a line of code which converts all your measurements into the metric system, displaying your output in kilograms and meters when you want it to use pounds and yards. You could remove that line of code so that the program only gives output in yards and pounds, and the revised program would run as if it had always been written that way. It won't "remember" that it used to calculate kilograms and meters, and experience any doubt about which system to use. The computer has no awareness or consciousness, and so it can't have any thoughts about how the program is running, nor about how it used to run before the correction. It just runs the program as currently written.

Not so with your brain! Your brain records thoughts as memories. While you can literally erase the computer code about the metric system and replace it with American measurements, your brain doesn't lose memories unless there has been actual physical damage to the brain. It creates new memories, and these memories can become the dominant memory on a subject, but you never lose the old memories. They may occur to you less often, even fall into disuse, but they can always become active again under the right circumstances.

Additionally, you have conscious awareness of thoughts as they occur in your cerebral cortex. This allows you to have thoughts about thoughts. Computers, at least to date (I hope my word processor doesn't have opinions about my writing), don't have this conscious awareness—they simply execute instructions without thinking about them.

Having thoughts about thoughts is what opens the door to worrying and arguing with yourself. Having thoughts about thoughts is what makes it so difficult to remove an "error of thinking" from your thoughts. Your effort to remove a thought will inevitably remind you of the thought you don't want to have. This is often typified in the classic, paradoxical instruction: "Don't think of a white bear."[1]

Paradoxical Therapy for Anxiety and Worry

A different school of psychotherapy which appeared about the same time as CBT was paradoxical therapy. This method didn't attain the same mainstream prominence that CBT has achieved but, in my opinion, can be a more powerful and direct way of working with chronic anxiety and worry. Paradoxical therapy takes a different approach to the problem of correcting your thoughts. It leaves thought alone and requests action instead. And it requests action in a paradoxical way, a request that is difficult to fully accept or reject.

A paradox is a seemingly logical request or instruction that leads to a self-contradictory result. A typical paradoxical request might be: "Be spontaneous now!" or "Listen carefully to what I say and don't do what I tell you." These kinds of instructions create confusion within the listener and make it difficult for her to keep doing the same old thing that she was doing before. "Act natural" is another example.

The principal tool of paradoxical therapy is called "prescribing the symptom." This has an astonishing amount of power in helping people overcome chronic anxiety. Here's an example of prescribing the symptom. When I work with a client who is struggling to overcome chronic worry, I might ask this person to deliberately keep her worries in mind as we have our conversation.

When I first do this, people have two principal reactions. First, they think I'm crazy, but I'll clear that up with them later. Second, they find it hard to keep that worry thought in mind and may find that they keep forgetting about their worry, even though I've asked them to pay more attention to it.

How does this work? My odd request for them to focus more on their worrisome thoughts interrupts and disrupts their internal effort to "stop worrying." And, it turns out, this effort to "stop worrying" is a major factor in maintaining chronic worry! When I disrupt it with my unexpected request, the worry actually becomes less persistent.

Paradoxical methods are powerful in working with chronic anxiety and worry because chronic anxiety is itself such a paradoxical experience. By that, I mean these two things:

1. Your efforts to directly increase anxiety will decrease it.

2. Your efforts to directly reduce anxiety will increase it.

In a larger sense, all the therapies mentioned above, including CBT, have a paradoxical aspect to them, because they all encourage the client to experience the anxiety in some way, to practice with it, in order to reduce it over time. This is why we invite the snake phobic to sit with a snake, the flying phobic to go for an airplane ride, the agoraphobic to go to the shopping mall, and so on. In my view, the elements of these therapies that encourage a person to work *with* the anxiety, rather than against, are the most powerful elements of those therapies. It's this paradoxical element of anxiety and worry that explains the observation "The harder I try, the worse it gets." It's the paradoxical element of anxiety that gives the Rule of Opposites its power.

CBT has been the treatment of choice for anxiety for the past thirty years. As its strengths and weaknesses have become more apparent, new ideas and models of how to work with anxious thoughts have appeared, including acceptance and commitment therapy, metacognitive therapy, dialectical behavior therapy, and narrative therapy, among others.

These models embody a different attitude toward thoughts than does traditional CBT. All these methods see thoughts as central in the production of emotions, but these newer methods take a much more skeptical attitude toward thoughts, and particularly toward our ability to control thoughts.

From this perspective, the brain produces thoughts in the same manner the kidneys produce urine and the liver produces bile. It's just what the organ does. And because you can only evaluate your thoughts with the same organ that produced those thoughts in the first place—your brain—you don't have a way to form an independent evaluation of your thoughts. None of us do. This is the reason people so often act as if their thoughts are a good, accurate model for the external world even when they're not.

This is also why we're so often attached to our thoughts, take pride in them as we would an important creation, and tend to find more value in our own thoughts than in anyone else's. So we have this problem, as expressed by Chicago comedian Emo Phillips: "I used to think that the brain was the most wonderful organ in my body. Then I realized who was telling me this."[2]

And we have the second problem that it isn't always so easy to directly change a thought. All too often the efforts people make to change their thoughts begin to work like thought stopping and, as I've previously noted, thought stopping is almost always unhelpful. The main result of "thought stopping" is "thought resumption."

If you use cognitive restructuring and find it helpful in modifying your worries without getting involved in a lot of arguing with yourself, without a lot of back talk from the worries, that's good. Keep doing that! However, if you find that you get bogged down in arguing with your thoughts when you seek to "correct" the errors, and that the worrisome thoughts continue to recur to you, then cognitive restructuring might be starting to work just like thought stopping for you. If that's the case, you may be better off using some of the acceptance-based techniques I present in chapters 8 to 10 rather than trying harder to make the cognitive restructuring work.

Acceptance and Commitment Therapy

Acceptance and commitment therapy has a lot to say about working with thoughts. ACT identifies thought and language as key sources of human misery. From this perspective, thought and language are the suitcase by which you can pack up your troubles and move from, say, New York to Los Angeles, yet experience the same thoughts and emotions in L.A. that you did in N.Y.

ACT identifies "cognitive fusion" as a principal problem.[3] What is cognitive fusion? It's when we give properties and characteristics to words and thoughts which only really belong to the objects those words describe.

What does that mean? Consider the example of a young child who gets scratched by the family cat. Young Susie may feel afraid of that cat for a while, might feel afraid of other cats and dogs in the neighborhood, might run from the room when a cat food commercial comes on television, and might even burst into tears or show signs of distress when someone mentions the word "cat." She can feel fear when she hears the word, even when the cat is outside. Susie has given the word "cat" the properties of scratchiness and "biteyness" that only actually belong to the animal. In ACT terms, she has "fused" the word "cat" with those properties. As a result, she can become afraid in the absence of the cat, just from hearing the word, or maybe even thinking the word. She no longer makes a distinction between hearing the word "cat" and seeing a cat leap at her, claws outspread.

As her parents notice this, they may try to help keep Susie calm by using some code to refer to "cat" when they find it necessary to mention that word in her presence. Maybe they use pig latin (ixnay with the atcay!) or refer to it as a banana rather than a cat. They're trying to care for Susie and protect her from upset. But they are also, unwittingly, strengthening the association Susie has formed between the sound of the word "cat" and those hurtful properties of "biteyness" and scratchiness, because they're depriving her of opportunities to get used to hearing the word.

Defusing "Hot Button" Words

You can see the same thing in anxiety and panic support groups all around the country, many of which discourage or prohibit the use of certain words that might bother their members. For instance, some support groups for people with panic attacks ask members to refrain from using the word "breathing" because some members are sensitive to this word and will have trouble catching their "b" if someone uses the "b" word! The group has fused the word "breathing" with the sensations of hyperventilation and all the symptoms that accompany it. Just as we saw with Susie and her parents, here we see people, intending to be kind and protective, acting in ways that lead people to feel more vulnerable, rather than less, to the "b" word.

Do you have some "hot button" words that you prefer to avoid, to skim over if you see them in print, words you don't want to say aloud because they might lead you to feel anxious?

You probably do, if you let your mind ponder it for a few moments. People with panic attacks often want to avoid words like "faint," "cerebral hemorrhage," "screaming insanity," and so on. People with social anxiety aren't so fond of words like "sweat," "tremble," and "blush." People with intrusive obsessive thoughts tend to avoid the key words from those thoughts, like "murder," "poison," "stab," "insecticide," and so on. Even people with just basic, garden variety anxiety have words that carry some special, "fused" feeling for them.

Want to try an experiment?

I hope by now you can guess where I'm going with this, and what the experiment is.

The experiment is: take one of those words and repeat it, out loud if you have the privacy to do that—twenty-five times.

If young Susie does that with the word "cat," the word will probably start to lose its claws.

By the way, if you did guess what the experiment would be, or something close, that's great—you're getting used to using the Rule of Opposites!

ACT seeks to help people undo this kind of cognitive fusion by fostering defusion—or as I call it, "de-fusion," since the technique aims to break the link you may have established between a word or thought and the actual properties you have come to associate with that thought. For instance, Susie's parents might help her to de-fuse the word "cat" from those properties of scratchiness and "biteyness" by making nonsense rhymes with the word cat, singing songs about cats, rhyming the word "cat," making artwork based on the word "cat," and so on. Panic support groups could help their members de-fuse the word "breathing" by similarly engaging in playful exercises that use, and overuse, the word.

De-fusion can be a powerful method by which you can reduce the misery you have come to feel in response to chronic worry. Misery often accompanies, for instance, disease, especially when it's a serious disease. However, people who struggle with chronic worry about disease can experience the same misery they associate with disease even when they are healthy, just from having thoughts about disease. That's why they tend to avoid watching medical shows on TV. They're trying to avoid anything that might remind them of disease. All that is necessary is to "fuse" the thought of disease with the misery of actually being ill. De-fusion is a method by which you can greatly reduce the amount of misery you experience in response to your unwanted thoughts.

ACT also seeks to help people spend more time in taking action with the external world around them and less time trying to rearrange or change the thoughts and feelings they experience in their internal world. In this sense, ACT has at least a superficial resemblance to the Serenity Prayer:

God, grant me the serenity to accept the things
    I cannot change,

The courage to change the things I can,

And the wisdom to know the difference.

When I received some ACT training, one of the general principles I took away was that it's probably more useful to help people examine how their thoughts influence their behavior than it is to spend time challenging the accuracy of the thoughts. (These characterizations of ACT and CBT are my own view and, while I think they're reasonably accurate, they represent how I use these methods, rather than how ACT and CBT experts may teach and use them.)

This represents perhaps the sharpest contrast between a traditional CBT or cognitive restructuring approach to thoughts and an ACT approach. Let's consider the example of a client who struggles with thoughts of being a coward. A CBT therapist would probably ask that client to define what he means by coward and then compare the client's behavior to that definition, taking note of when the client acted like a coward and when he did not. In this way, the therapist would help the client to get a more balanced and accurate view of his behavior with the ultimate goal of helping the client to achieve more accuracy in his thoughts.

An ACT therapist, on the other hand, isn't going to get involved in looking at the accuracy, or lack thereof, of that thought about being a coward at all. An ACT therapist is more likely to ask a question like this: "This thought you have about being a coward—is it getting in the way of you doing anything that's important to you?"

In other words, an ACT therapist will help you look at your thoughts in terms of how they influence your behavior, rather than how accurate or inaccurate they may be. The implicit goal is to help you to behave, in the external world, more in keeping with your own hopes and aspirations for your life rather than being limited by whatever thoughts happen to crop up in your internal world.

Twists and Turns: How Thoughts Can Affect Behavior

I happened to be working with a client who was continually worrying about his retirement plan around the time I was first learning about ACT. This man wasn't close to retirement, nor did he have any financial problems. In fact, he was relatively well off. But he was obsessively preoccupied with this worrisome thought: *What if my retirement plan turns out to be insufficient by the time I retire?* This worrisome thought, and his ongoing efforts to rid himself of this thought, were his near-constant companions, and he used all the anti-worry responses we looked at in chapter 3, with little benefit.

He and I worked cognitive restructuring really hard. We looked at his thoughts about how terrible retirement might be if he had less money than anticipated. We reviewed the options he would have then to cut back his expenses and considered how those lifestyle changes might affect his mood and thoughts. We considered cutbacks he could make in his current spending patterns in order to give him a higher probability of a solid retirement income, and how he would think and feel about that set of changes. We reviewed his thoughts about working part time in retirement, should he feel that necessary, and the possibility of his spouse playing a large role in moneymaking. He found neither comfort nor reduction in worry from these efforts.

I suggested the potential benefits of getting an expert review of his plan from a financial planner, only to learn that he had already done this several times. The problem he experienced with this attempted solution was that, when you consult a financial planner, they typically want you to sign a document acknowledging that their forecasts are built on certain assumptions which might not turn out to be accurate, and promising you won't sue them for that. "Not accurate?" he said. "That was why I went there in the first place, to get an accurate prediction!"

We were getting nowhere slowly! One day it occurred to me that an ACT therapist wouldn't be doing all this work of looking at how true or false his worries about retirement were. I remembered the ACT question, "Is having this thought getting in the way of you doing anything important?" And so I asked him that question.

It turned out it *was* getting in the way of him doing something important, and when I heard what it was, I realized immediately that I had misunderstood the problem. You can try to guess what it was before I tell you, but I doubt anyone will guess it correctly.

It wasn't preventing him from working, or retiring, or saving money. It was preventing him from doing something else, something that made me realize I had been approaching the wrong problem.

What was it? When you belong to a retirement plan, either on your own or through an employer, you get a periodic report about how your plan is doing. It shows the contributions you've made; the contributions your employer's made, if any; and the change in the market value of your stock and bond holdings in the plan. This is the information people use to monitor and change their investment strategy as needed.

This man's worrisome thoughts prevented him from opening the retirement report when it came in the mail. He would put it in a filing cabinet unopened.

I realized then that I had misdiagnosed the problem. I had been proceeding as if this man needed to feel more secure in his financial planning. But now I could see that he was so intolerant of worry and uncertainty that he was willing to give up control of his finances, if only that would relieve his worry!

He didn't need to become more confident and sure—he needed to become *more willing to feel unsure*, and live with that set of thoughts and feelings. He needed to do more work *with* the worry, and less against.

Thinking It Over

Thinking about your worries, in an effort to evaluate and correct them, has some limitations, and these limitations may hamper your effort to calm worrisome thoughts with cognitive restructuring.

For one thing, thinking objectively about your thoughts is quite difficult, maybe impossible, because the tool you use to evaluate your thoughts—your brain—is the same tool that created them in the first place. For another, your efforts to evaluate and correct your worrisome thoughts will often produce a kind of internal arguing with your thoughts, rather than the calm resolution that you originally hoped for.

If you find that these limitations hamper your efforts to reduce chronic worry with cognitive restructuring, you might find more relief with the techniques of cognitive de-fusion. Working with (rather than against) the key words and thoughts of your chronic worry, particularly in a playful, humorous manner, may well give you better results than efforts to rationalize and correct the content of your worries.

Uncle Argument and Your Relationship with Worry

How are you doing with the Tic Tacs from chapter 6? It's often surprising to see how thoroughly this "what if" habit has infiltrated your daily thoughts. I encourage you to continue using the Tic Tacs for a few weeks, because this will help you build your ability to observe, as if from a distance, your own worry habits and invitations.

This chapter will lay out the big picture of what a good relationship with worry looks like and offer some specific steps you can take to start traveling that path. Approach this the same way you would approach any significant lifestyle change like diet or exercise—focus on taking the steps and building them into your daily life rather than looking for immediate success. It's understandable that people look for quick results when making a change, but all too often that focus on quick results detracts from their ability to stay on path with the new habit. The key here is to build the new habits into your life and then, over time, reap the benefits.

Here's a phrase that can help you keep this in mind: *Feelings follow behavior.* Be it a diet, an exercise plan, or a worry reduction program, we all want to feel good as soon as possible. But the good feelings will likely come after, not before, we make the changes in our habits and daily routine.

What's a Good Relationship with Worry?

Let's suppose you're going to a family event. Maybe it's a wedding, a graduation party, a bar mitzvah, or a fiftieth anniversary party. You're looking forward to it and want to enjoy it. Unfortunately, you misplaced the invitation for a while. You were the last person to send in your RSVP, and so they seated you next to Uncle Argument at the banquet table.

Uncle Argument is actually an okay person, but he really, really likes to argue. That's pretty much his entire conversational style. If you're a Democrat, he's a Republican. If you think American football is the greatest sport, he picks soccer. If you think breakfast is the most important meal, he says that it's dinner, and so on. The man just loves to argue. He's not really mean, he just loves arguing.

And you'll be seated next to him at dinner. You don't want to argue. You want to sit and eat, you want to enjoy the meal, you want to have some pleasant conversation if possible, but you absolutely don't want to argue. Arguing gives you a stomachache. What can you do?

It's Hard to Avoid Arguing

You can't move to another table, because there aren't any empty seats. You can't change seats with anybody, because nobody wants to sit next to Uncle Argument. So you have to sit next to him unless you skip the meal. You don't want to do that because that's usually the part you enjoy the most, and going without food gives you a stomachache as well. How can you sit next to Uncle Argument for the entire meal without arguing? What would your options be?

You might try ignoring him, but that just makes him louder and more persistent. He loves it when people try to ignore him, because he takes that to mean he's winning the argument. So that won't help.

You might tell him you don't want to argue, but that also makes him more persistent, and he'll start nagging you about being afraid to voice your opinion. You could yell at him, tell him to shut up, but that's angry arguing, which delights and encourages him. You could listen carefully for him to say something that's clearly wrong, and then point that out to him, but that's also arguing, and he never admits to being wrong anyway. You could try to get other people at the table to help you out, but they don't want to mess with Uncle Argument, so they'll look the other way. You're on your own!

You could hit him, but you probably won't get invited to the next family event if you start a fistfight at this one. And you don't want to bring the police to the party. So what can you do?

The Opposite of Arguing

How about this—you can humor him. You can agree with everything he says, true or untrue, brilliant or ridiculous, whatever. "Yes, Uncle Argument, how very true. So wise. From your mouth to God's ears."

Do you have any doubt that if you agree with everything he says, this man who loves arguing more than anything else will find someone else to argue with? Do you give anything up by humoring him? Would this be a reasonable way of responding to the persistent invitation to argue?

You can have an arguing, confrontational relationship with him, or you can have a humoring relationship with him. The man is so persistent that he leaves you no other choice. You wish you had other choices, but you also want to enjoy the banquet, and these are the choices you have.

Dealing with your worry is like dealing with Uncle Argument. If you take the bait and reply to the specific content of the arguments, you end up getting embroiled when you just wanted to eat. You end up exactly where you didn't want to be—arguing, and finding that your comfort level is decreasing.

On the other hand, if you create the habit of humoring your worrisome thoughts, you can increasingly pass over the invitation to argue without becoming embroiled or upset. You can play with the thoughts, rather than work against them.

Does this sound counterintuitive? That's good, because the problem *is* counterintuitive. If it's true that the harder you try to suppress these thoughts, the worse they get, then you will probably benefit from trying something very different. Humoring the thoughts will be just what the Rule of Opposites would suggest.

Is That Okay with You?

Do you have any objections to this? Sometimes people express some reservations in the form of "should" statements, as in, "He"—Uncle Argument—"should be more respectful of my feelings" and "I shouldn't have to deal with all these stupid thoughts!" But if that were going to get you somewhere, you'd be sitting at a lovely café without a care in the world, while a beautiful stranger reads poetry to you, instead of reading this book. Better to work with "what is" than to get stressed about those thoughts of what "should be."

A New Way to Look at Worry

This "Uncle Argument" metaphor might be very different from the ways you've thought about chronic worry in the past. How have you thought about your chronic worry in the past? What kind of metaphors come to mind?

Most people who struggle with chronic worry tend to use metaphors that involve struggle, resistance, and fighting. They may think about the anxiety demon and how they can slay it. It's natural enough to think about chronic worry in terms of demonizing it and opposing it. That's a very intuitive response.

But this is a counterintuitive problem…and so when we rely on our natural intuitive responses, we often end up feeling frustrated in our attempts to solve a problem. When I'm skidding on an icy road, the harder I try to steer away from that phone pole, the more likely I am to hit it. I need to steer *into* the skid.

So it is with our metaphors for chronic worry. Worry is not a disease or a soul-sucking alien that's invaded my mind. It's just the natural consequence of my brain looking out for me, probably more than necessary. A counterintuitive response is much more likely to get me where I want to be. That will take a little getting used to.

Worry Is Like a Heckler

Chronic worry is like a heckler in the audience at a performance. Dealing with a heckler requires a particular kind of response. As a performer, it won't help to go down into the audience and have a fistfight with the heckler, because that prevents you from delivering the performance you came for. Neither will it help to defend yourself against the heckler's comments, because then you're arguing with the heckler rather than doing your show. And it won't do to try and ignore the heckling either, because it will be noticeable no matter how hard you try not to notice, and struggling not to notice will distract you from the task at hand. You could perhaps ask the heckler to stop, but generally speaking, hecklers don't respond to simple requests to be reasonable. Your request will probably fall on deaf ears and the heckling will continue, and meanwhile you've again been distracted from your task.

What's a good way to respond to a heckler? It's probably best to work the heckler into your routine. This way, you don't have to choose between going on with your show (or daily business) and listening to the heckler. And, as you work with the heckling in this way, treating it like you would any other sounds in the room, the heckling will probably die down. What keeps heckling going is the sense that the heckling is getting attention and being disruptive. As it starts to blend in with the show, it will probably diminish.

Are You Being Heckled By Your Own Thoughts?

What does it mean when you find yourself getting heckled by your own thoughts? As we saw in chapter 4, it means you're nervous. That's probably all it means—not endangered, just nervous. You could run a quick check with the two-part test from chapter 2 if you want.

Suppose you get an e-mail from a Nigerian prince, in which he offers to share a fortune in gold with you. He just needs you to give him access to your bank account so he can transfer it to you.

If you take the content of this e-mail at face value—if you take it to mean that you'll soon be rich—you're going to get suckered. However, if you read the content of the e-mail and make an interpretation of what it means—that someone is trying to scam you—you'll probably come out of it all right.

These worrisome thoughts (the heckling) need to be interpreted in a similar way. The repetitive "what if" thoughts don't really, accurately predict illness, job loss, boiler failure, kids flunking out of school, and so on. What they do mean is "I'm nervous."

And that's what you have to respond to—nervousness, not disaster.

Humoring the Worry

So how about doing some humoring? There are a lot of ways to do this. Here's one method.

Simply take the thought, accept it, and exaggerate it. There's a training exercise in improvisational theater called "Yes, and…" In this exercise, you accept whatever the other person in the scene has just told you, and build on it by adding something else. You don't disagree, or contradict, or deny what the other player just said. You accept it and add to it. This is probably the most fundamental rule of improvisational comedy—no denial! Instead, accept whatever the other performers offer you and build on it.

This rule works on stage and will also work in your own mind, in your internal world. The reason it works so well on stage is different from the reason it works so well with worry, but this rule definitely helps with worry. It helps because it's an expression of the Rule of Opposites.

How can you use it? Here are some examples of humoring the thoughts in this way.

What if I freak out on the airplane and they have to restrain me?

Yes, and when the plane lands they'll probably parade me through town before taking me to the asylum, and I'll be on the nightly news for everyone to see.

What if I get so nervous at the banquet that my hands shake so everyone can see?

Yes, and I'll probably spill hot soup all over the bridal party and cause second degree burns, so the honeymoon will be ruined.

What if I get a fatal illness?

Yes, and I better call the hospital to make a reservation now, and probably the funeral home, too.

The point of this response is not to get rid of the worry. My clients are often so used to trying to rid themselves of their chronic worry that they'll sometimes try the humoring response for a while, then come back to me and say "It didn't work. I still worry." That's *not* the aim of humoring.

Worry is counterintuitive. When you try to remove it, by whatever means, it becomes more persistent. The point of a humoring response is to become more accepting of the worry so that it matters less to you. It's to get better at hearing and accepting the thought for what it is—simply a thought, a twitch in your internal world. It's okay to have thoughts—smart ones, dumb ones, pleasant ones, angry ones, scary ones, and so on. We don't have that much choice in the matter. We all have lots of thoughts. And a lot of them are misleading and exaggerated. That's okay. We don't have to be guided by them, or argue with them, or disprove them, or silence them. We just have to be willing to hear them as we go on about our business.

I notice that my clients with chronic worry go through a cycle. When they have a time of extra worry, they label it "a bad time" and struggle to bring it to an end. When they have a time of reduced worry, they label it "a good time" and try to keep the worry at bay. They're always trying to adjust their menu of thoughts—and it usually brings a very different result than they intended.

What's a person to do? When you try to get rid of the "bad times," it often prolongs and strengthens them. When you try to hold on to the "good times," they get ripped from your hands.

Frustrating, right? Let's recall that important observation: *The harder I try, the worse it gets.* How can you apply that here?

You might identify your worry thought and "keep that thought in mind." What does that mean, to keep that thought in mind? It means the opposite of what you do when you try to "keep that thought *out* of mind!" You deliberately keep the thought at hand, playing with it, repeating it, trying not to forget about it, maybe checking in with yourself every three minutes or so to make sure you remember to repeat the thought to yourself periodically.

Why would anyone do that? Well, if it's true that "the harder I try, the worse it gets," you'll probably get better results doing the *opposite* of what you usually do!

Become Less Attached to Your Thoughts

Another good way, a more general one, and perhaps the most important of all, is to get less attached to your thoughts, regardless of whether the content of those thoughts seems good or bad. Your automatic thoughts are like an unending soundtrack that accompanies you your entire life. Sometimes the thoughts are relevant, sometimes not; sometimes pleasant, sometimes not; sometimes accurate, sometimes not. There's no off switch, no volume control. We live in our thoughts the same way a goldfish lives in water.

Neither you nor I get to pick our thoughts. We can, however, often pick how we respond to them, and we can certainly pick what we do with our time on this planet. We don't need to get our thoughts arranged the way we might like in order to do things we want to do.

This work that people do of trying to hold onto the "good" thoughts and get rid of the "bad" thoughts—where do they do it? In their heads! As the activity of life goes on around them, they're missing out, because they're inside, trying once again to rearrange the furniture rather than coming out here into the sunlight where life actually occurs. Let your thoughts come and go in your head while you tend to the activities that are important to you out in the external world, the environment of people and objects that you live in.

Want to try an experiment? It won't take long, maybe five minutes. It's got three steps.

The Worry Experiment

Step One. Create a sentence, maximum of twenty-five words, that expresses the strongest version you can create of one of your typical worries, something that's been bothering you recently. The first two words, of course, will be "what if," so you really only have twenty-three words to play with. Try to create a thought that not only includes the terrible event you fear but also incorporates the long-term consequences of this problem, the angst you'll feel in your old age as you remember this bad event, and so on. This will be the longest of the three steps. Spend some time on it to get a good worry expression and to get the most unpleasant ideas in it that you can.

Here are a couple of examples. As you might expect, simply reading these examples of worry will induce discomfort in many readers, the same way a scary book or movie will fill a person with fear. That's okay, it will pass. However, if you don't feel up to that experience right now, bookmark this section and come back some other time when you're more willing to feel that discomfort.

Examples:

For someone who worries about losing his/her sanity:

WEAK: *What if I go crazy?*

BETTER: *What if I go crazy and end up in an institution?*

GOOD: *What if I go crazy, end up in an institution, and live a long, miserable, pointless life—forgotten, toothless, with bad hair, abandoned and alone?*

For someone who worries about looking foolish at a party:

WEAK: *What if I get really nervous at the party?*

BETTER: *What if I get really nervous at the party, and then start sweating and trembling?*

GOOD: *What if I get really nervous at the party, start sweating and trembling, pee in my pants, and people avoid me the rest of my life?*

Go ahead and draft your worry. Use a topic that you usually find quite upsetting, in order to make this experiment meaningful. State the "what if" worry and add two or three "and then" statements of the terrible consequences it will produce. Don't just stop with your first draft. Take a little time to edit it and get the maximum strength—all the fear and loathing you can muster—into your wording.

Step Two. Write the numbers one to twenty-five on a slip of paper.

Step Three. Sit, or stand, in front of a mirror so you can see yourself. Say the worry sentence out loud, slowly, twenty-five times. After each repetition, cross off the next number on your slip of paper, so you can keep count.

If you prefer, you can group twenty-five small items—toothpicks, coins, jellybeans (or Tic Tacs!)—on a table, moving them one at a time with each repetition. Don't count in your head, because that takes too much concentration. I want you to concentrate on the twenty-five repetitions of the worrisome thought.

Go ahead and try this. Pick a time and place that allows you privacy, so you can focus your attention on what you're saying without a lot of concern for being overheard. You may feel foolish anyway, but please do give it a fair try. Don't skip past this!

This exercise may not be a pleasant experience, but I think it will be worth the temporary pain. Experiments like this one will be very helpful in developing a better understanding of how your worry works and in cultivating a different way of responding to it. Come back when you're done.

It seems odd and counterintuitive, this idea, but remember what kind of results you've obtained from logical and intuitive efforts in the past. Just check it out—it's an experiment!

All done? So now, if you were doing this experiment in my office, the question I would ask is this: How did the emotional impact of the last repetition compare to the emotional impact of the first repetition? Which one bothered you more?

Repeating the Worry Usually Reduces Its Power!

If you're like most people with chronic worry, you probably found that the worrisome thought *lost* power with repetition, so that the last repetition felt much less disturbing than the first one. And if you did, this offers a powerful insight into the nature of your chronic worry. (If you didn't get this result, review the worry you used to make sure it's representative of your chronic worries, and replace it if it's not. If it is a representative statement, you might be dealing with a different kind of problem—depressive memories of a past event, rather than worrisome thoughts of a possible future event, for instance; or a strong obsessive compulsive tendency. If this is the case, perhaps you should review your work with the earlier chapters, or review your situation with a professional therapist skilled in this type of work.)

Think of all the efforts you've made to rid yourself of the worry, and how little you have to show for them. Think of the results you've obtained from the anti-worry techniques you listed in chapter 3. Yet here, with just a few moments of repeating your worry out loud, you probably reduced its ability to disturb you—not permanently, of course, but the repetition produced a temporary change in your emotional response to the worry.

"What if" this is more like the way to respond to chronic worry? "What if" this approach—humoring and making plenty of room for the worry—has more to offer you than all the thought stopping methods you've heard so much about?

This would mean a major revision of your relationship with chronic worry. It would suggest a counterintuitive response to a counterintuitive problem. Consistent with the Rule of

Opposites, you would respond to chronic worry by accepting and playing with the thoughts, rather than trying to rid yourself of them. You would defuse the worry thoughts by accepting them as sources of doubt, rather than danger. You would humor the worries, rather than get drawn into unwanted argument. You would treat them like a tic, rather than a tumor.

In short, you can replace the counterproductive thought stopping with the very productive thought exposure. A snake phobic who wants to overcome that phobia will need to spend some time with snakes in order to overcome the fear. If you have an ongoing issue with chronic worry, the worrisome thoughts are your snakes.

I've worked with clients who feared snakes and wanted to overcome that fear, and I've done that by having one or more extended exposure sessions with a client and a snake. While the problem initially seems insurmountable to the client, it's not really a hard job to help them overcome it. I just have to take the time to help them accept the symptoms of fear and get involved with the snake. The desensitization to the snake then occurs quite naturally.

The only thing I have to remember is to get a nonpoisonous snake. And with chronic worry, all the snakes are nonpoisonous. Thoughts, however upsetting, foul, disgusting, annoying, and so on, are just never dangerous. It's discomfort, not danger.

For some people, it will be enough to take the humoring response as I've described it here. If you can do that, and return your energy and attention back to the activities that are important to you, that might be all that you need to do.

Other people may find the habit of chronic worry more persistent and entrenched in their lives and will benefit from using more specific and tailored techniques. You'll find those in the next chapter.

Thinking It Over

In this chapter, we've looked at a basic tool you can use to shift your relationship with chronic worry in a helpful direction. You tried an experiment of repeating worrisome thoughts to evaluate what happens if you make room for the thoughts, rather than resist them. And we looked at ways you can humor these thoughts, the same way you might humor Uncle Argument. In chapter 9, we'll look at more active ways you can respond to particularly persistent and unpleasant thoughts.

AHA! Three Steps for Handling Chronic Worry

Here's your proverbial AHA! moment in dealing with worry. This is an acronym you can use to help you remember a couple of steps to take when you're being bothered by worrisome thoughts.

Acknowledge and accept.

Humor *the worrisome thoughts, as you would humor Uncle Argument.*

Activity—*resume doing things that are important to you in your "external world" (and take the worries with you if necessary).*

Here's a detailed explanation for each step of AHA!

Acknowledge and Accept

What's to acknowledge here? That you're having a worrisome thought, once again! It might be annoying to find it back in your head. You might want to refuse to acknowledge its appearance because it seems so unreasonable that, once again, this thought is occurring to you. It offers nothing of value, and you've dismissed it so many times before, yet here it is again, serving no useful purpose, bothering you like a spam e-mail that shows up in your mailbox every hour. Or maybe, even though you've had lots of experiences with these worrisome thoughts and have never been harmed by them, you still respond with fear because you wonder, *What if this is the time that something happens?* and you get tricked by that thought into taking the content seriously. You wish you could be perfectly sure that the thought is false, for all time, but of course you can't have that certainty.

So, okay—you can simply acknowledge that you're having another occurrence of a worrisome thought. Maybe you recognized it by the "what if" introduction, or maybe you didn't catch on until you considered the content it was offering you, but okay. You have a brain, so you have thoughts. No need to try to ignore it, or pretend it's not there. There's nothing wrong with ignoring it, really—but if the effort you make to ignore the thought keeps bringing it back to your attention, then trying to ignore the thought isn't helping. Here you are, having another one of the many, many thoughts you will have today, and this one happens to be a loser.

Whom do you acknowledge it to? Usually just yourself. This is an internal process in which you briefly notice the presence of the worrisome thoughts, acknowledge them without resistance or suppression, and move on to the next thing. Sometimes you might have reasons to mention the worrisome thoughts to others, and we'll take a look at that in chapter 12.

What's to accept? The fact that you're having a thought you don't like! You may or may not agree with the content of the thought. You may find it reasonable or you might find it repulsive. It doesn't really matter! You don't get to pick and choose which thoughts you'll have and which thoughts you won't have—nobody does! There's no need to try to contradict the thought, to disprove it, to make it go away, or to reassure yourself. There probably won't be any benefit if you do.

No one expects you to control your thoughts. You're accountable for your actions, and you'll be judged by your actions. Not by thoughts! You can have a worrisome thought, same as you can have an angry thought, a jealous thought, a sexy thought, a wacky thought, a kind thought, an unkind thought, a shameful thought, a compassionate thought, a murderous thought, or whatever. To say that worries are a dime a dozen would be to greatly exaggerate their value.

So, okay—you can allow yourself to have whatever thoughts happen to come to mind, same as you'll allow yourself to have whatever noises your stomach might make, same as you'll allow yourself to have whatever reactions you might have to an unpleasant odor. If someone else hears your stomach grumble and you feel embarrassed, you can go ahead and say "excuse me" if you wish. No one can hear your thought, so there's no occasion for apology; you don't control your thoughts, so there's no need for judgment. Here you are, having a thought that you wouldn't choose to have, if you could make the choice. Which you can't.

Recently a client, who tends to be a little perfectionistic and demanding of herself, asked me, "But what can I say to myself when I notice I'm having one of these thoughts again?" I suggested, "Oh well." She had thought something more complicated, more powerful and cleansing would be necessary. Nope! This is not, as the saying goes, rocket science. *You don't control your thoughts, nor do your thoughts control you.* When it comes to automatic thoughts like these, you're more like the reader of a book than you are like the author, so no need to engage in a prideful struggle to control your thoughts. You don't get to pick the thoughts you have or exclude the thoughts you think should be excluded. Oh well! When I get to design the world, there'll be some changes made!

This first step—acknowledge and accept—is probably the most important and powerful of the three. I describe it as simply as possible, but that doesn't mean it's easy. Some people may be able to simply acknowledge and accept the unwanted thoughts and move on to the activity step without the use of any other techniques or responses. That's great! If that works for you, just move on without spending any time on this step.

That tends to be the exception, though. Most people find that the thoughts are a little "stickier" than that, that they can't move on so quickly because they find that they're still arguing with Uncle Argument, still wishing the thought would cease and desist. Cultivating an accepting attitude toward thoughts you detest and fear is usually a long, gradual process, a task we work on all our lives rather than a specific goal we attain quickly and completely. It's something that you practice and acquire over time, not something that you simply "do."

It reminds me of the slogan on the box of the Othello board game. Othello is a deceptively simple game with pieces like checkers, with a black side and a white side. You win by out-flanking your opponent's pieces and flipping them over to your color. Sounds simple, but the game is actually quite complex, and the slogan is "a minute to learn, a lifetime to master."

If you became dehydrated, perhaps because you played too much tennis on a hot, sunny day without adequate liquids, you could drink more water and solve the problem. If you were severely dehydrated, you might require intravenous fluids. That's all it would take—resupply your fluids and the problem is fixed.

Training yourself to handle your worrisome thoughts differently is not like the problem of resupplying your water. It's more like the process of exercising to get yourself back into shape, or of dieting and losing weight. You will need to learn, practice, and continually follow some steps in order to improve and get the results you seek.

What's most important about dieting is acquiring, and following, the habit of eating a healthy menu each day and getting regular exercise. That's more important than whatever you happen to weigh today, because if you continue with your good habits, your weight and physical condition will generally fall into line. In the same way, what's most important here is acquiring a regular habit of how you respond to worrisome thoughts, not how many worrisome thoughts you have today. What's really important is moving in the right direction. It's much less important how fast you go, or how gracefully.

In order to figure out some good ways to respond to a worry, first clarify the kind of situation you confront now. You can do this by using the two-part test from chapter 2, which asks:

1. Is there a problem that exists now in the external world around you?

2. If there is, can you do something to change it now?

If you get anything other than two "yes" answers—two "no" answers, one "no" and one "yes," maybes, or whatever—then you don't have a problem in your external world that you can solve right now. You have the problem of worrying. You're being "baited" by Uncle Argument.

The experience of getting baited and bothered by worrisome thoughts is similar to what you see if you hold up a small mirror to an aquarium containing a Siamese fighting fish. These fish are kept alone because the males fight to the death if they're housed together. When I was a kid, we would hold up a mirror and watch the fearsome display this fish would put on when he saw himself. Thinking the image was another fish, our fish would prepare for combat, turning a bright red with gills out, fins waving, mouth opening wide, and so on. Of course, there wasn't any other fish to fight, and after a while the fish would calm down; but for a few minutes he'd get really riled up, the same way you might if bothered by a worrisome thought. The reaction is real. The threat is not. It's a fake fish!

When this happens, keep two points in mind. It might help to put these on your electronic device or a 3 by 5 card until you get in the habit of remembering.

1. What you have is the emotion of feeling nervous.

2. It's okay to feel nervous. You probably really, really dislike the emotion, but it's like the experience of sitting in an uncomfortably warm room, not like camping in a forest fire. It's discomfort, not danger. You might be sitting in an uncomfortably warm room and reading about a forest fire, or watching a movie about a forest fire, but it's still just discomfort, no matter how realistic the film is or how vivid the description.

The problem you face is not the problem described in the catastrophe clause of your worry. The problem you face is the discomfort you experience in response to the worrisome thought, and your natural inclination to take that thought seriously and resist it. When you resist the thought with your usual selection of anti-worry responses, this is when you once again experience the difficulty of *The harder I try, the worse it gets.*

That's the first step, acknowledge and accept. If you find that you frequently take the bait and get caught up in arguing with Uncle Argument, then this second step will be probably be helpful.

Humor the Worrisome Thoughts

Having acknowledged the temporary presence of the thought, and accepted its presence as best you can, you might now find it helpful to respond to the worrisome thought in a playful, counterintuitive style.

So do something very different. Employ the Rule of Opposites. Here are some ways you can respond, in a playful or silly manner, to the problem of getting "hooked" by Uncle Argument's efforts to get you embroiled.

Sing a worry song. You can make a song of your worry. I have some examples of this on my website, songs about panic attacks, sung in my own dreadful voice. Pick a catchy tune that's easy to sing to, and create your own worrisome lyrics about the disasters that are waiting for you around every corner.

Here, for instance, is the first verse of one of my songs about panic attacks. It's sung to the tune of "Camptown Races":

I'll go crazy, then I'll die

Doo dah, doo dah

Panic gonna get me by and by

Oh, doo dah day

Make my head feel light

Make my heart race all day

Run stark naked through shopping malls

Doo dah, doo dah day

Write a haiku. If you don't feel like singing, you can write a haiku. Haiku is a traditional Japanese poetry form. There's a lot to learn about haiku, but for our purposes we'll just focus on one simplistic aspect of it.

It's a three-line poem, without rhymes. The first line is five syllables. The second is seven. The third is five. You simply write a three-line unrhymed poem of your worries that fits this format.

Let's suppose you have a bothersome thought and recognize it for what it is, but still can't simply dismiss it. You've tried to reason your way out of it and you've tried to distract yourself. Your usual ways of interrupting the thought don't seem to be working for you. You're still trying to fight the fake fish! This would be a good time to haiku.

Here are some haikus I've received.

I feel dizzy now.

I'll probably go insane.

Please water my plants.

I'm on the plane now.

They will see me shake and cry.

Please pass the barf bags.

If haiku is a little too exotic for you, how about a limerick?

Write a limerick. A limerick is a five-line poem that you probably first encountered when you were a child. The first, second, and fifth lines rhyme with each other and have the same number of syllables (usually eight or nine). The third and fourth lines rhyme with each other and have the same number of syllables (usually five or six). This structure sounds complicated, but it's easier than it sounds! And it gives a limerick its characteristic rhythm. Limericks often start with the line "There once was a…" or "There was a…"

Here's a sample limerick.

A woman from near Cincinnati

Thought, *What if I turn out real batty?*

It'll ruin my brain

They'll declare me insane

And my friends will all be so catty

Worry in your second language. Are you bilingual? Even if you just have high school training in a second language, that might be enough to enable you to do your worrying in your second language.

Or, if you don't know a second language at all, you can use pig latin. Pig latin is just a simple way to transform English words into something that sounds quite different. Parents use it to talk in front of their children about topics they want to keep secret.

There are two rules to basic pig latin. For words starting with consonants (or consonant clusters), move the consonant to the end of the word, followed by "ay." For words starting with vowels, simply add "ay" to the end of the word. There are a few other rules for special cases, and you can find those on the Internet if you want. So, for instance:

What if I freak out? atWhay ifyay Iyay eakfray outyay?

What if I left the stove on? atWhay ifyay Iyay eftlay ethay ovestay onyay?

As with haiku and limericks, we're not changing the content of the worry thoughts here. We're just changing the format, and that can really change your response to the worry. When you try to remember how you might say "choke to death" in German, it often produces a very different result!

Worry in a fake foreign accent. Yes, it's silly, but why not? Silly can help you keep a good perspective on the worry. No need to give the worry content more respect than it deserves.

List your worries. Make a list of your chronic worries. Start with a basic list of the ones that frequently occur to you, and add to it over time as you notice new ones. Once you have the basic list, you can get into the habit, each time you notice a worry, of quickly checking to see if it's on your list. If it's not, add it. Once you see it on your list, go on about your business, secure in the knowledge that you have recorded this worry and can return to it at any time. You don't have to keep thinking about it right now, because it's recorded on your list.

This list will be useful when you work with the exercise I'll discuss in chapter 10.

Record your worries. You can make audio recordings of your worries, on your smart phone or other digital device. The idea here is to mimic the process that occurs in your head as you worry. This usually involves a lot of repetition of a couple of simple "what if" thoughts.

There are several ways to do this. One is to make a short recording, perhaps thirty to sixty seconds, of a single "what if" worry. Say it several times, as many as will fit in the short recording. You can then set aside times during the day—ten-minute periods—when you can set the device to continually play and replay the recorded worry. The effect is similar to what you would get if you could eavesdrop on someone's thoughts while they were engaged in worry.

People are often concerned that if they do this, the worry will somehow become more compelling, and they will be unable to stop. However, think back to the experiment with the twenty-five repetitions in chapter 8—hopefully you did that experiment—and be guided by the results you got with it. When people do that experiment, they almost always find the worry loses its emotional punch and hold on their attention as they do more repetitions.

Another way to use recordings is to record a longer worry session, one that's more like an argument with Uncle Argument, in which you go back and forth with the worry, trying to disprove it, to silence it, to calm it, and so on. Play both parts of the argument—Uncle Argument as he tries to get your goat, and you as you try to calm and reassure yourself. You might want to make a recording of thirty minutes with this approach, and set aside time to listen to it regularly.

Do You Worry about Playing with Worries?

These suggestions are probably very different from what you've been trying. They involve accepting and playing with your worrisome thoughts rather than resisting and taking them seriously.

What reactions do you have to the idea of humoring your chronic worry?

People are often nervous at first about humoring their worrisome thoughts. It seems risky to them, like they're tempting fate. They may have certain beliefs about worry that suggest the worry needs to be treated very seriously, and carefully, as if chronic worry were itself dangerous. I'll take a look at some of these beliefs in chapter 11.

If you prefer to treat these worries more formally, you can use the Worry Journal that's available on the New Harbinger website (http://www.newharbinger.com/33186). It's simply a questionnaire you can use *while* you are caught up in the worries. Take a little time to observe your worries, and answer the questions listed in the Journal. This will train you to be a better observer of your worrisome thoughts and will help you detach from arguing and resisting. If a bull simply observed with interest the antics of the bullfighter with the red cape, there wouldn't be any gory bullfights!

The Worry Journal can be quite helpful. However, I encourage you to experiment with the more humorous, playful responses as well, because I think they will bring you greater rewards over the long run.

When are you done with this second step? Don't keep repeatedly humoring the worry, again and again, waiting for it to go away. That's too much like arguing with Uncle Argument! Instead, take a humoring stance with the thoughts and then move on to the third step, allowing them to follow you as you get back into the external world, if that's what they do.

Activity—Resume Doing Things That Are Important to You (and Take the Worries with You If Necessary)

If you've ever had an eye exam, you're probably familiar with the part where the doctor switches through pairs of lenses, asking you "Better here...or better here?" while you try to decide which lens gives you better vision.

You face a similar choice when you're caught up in worry. The choice is this: "Better here (in your internal world of worry)...or better here (in your external world)?"

It's generally much more helpful to get involved in the external world. It's better to engage in activities that are usually important or fun for you, while you're worried and uncomfortable, than it is to spend much time in your head, trying to get rid of the thoughts. The reason external involvement is a better choice is *not* because you will feel better right away; you might not. But it will lead to a better outcome and a better pattern for the future.

When I take a group of fearful fliers on a flight, there are often one or two people who have a terribly hard time boarding the plane. They stand in the gate, trying so hard to get more comfortable with the idea of boarding, but they can't find the comfort they want, and so they feel stuck.

If they make their choice on the basis of wanting to feel better right away, they walk away and go home. They do feel better immediately, but it doesn't last. By the time they get to the parking lot they start feeling regret, and they have a pretty miserable rest of the day. On the other hand, if they decide on the basis of how they want to feel, not right then but that night, then they get on the plane, feeling afraid in the moment, because they know they'll feel real good when they return home with that accomplishment behind them.

You face a similar choice with worry. It's tempting to figure that you should do a little more thinking about the thoughts, to try again to review them or reason with them in an effort to feel better right now, but that's a shell game. You won't win that game because it's rigged against you. It's for suckers! The Rule of Opposites suggests, well, the opposite. Let's go do something else while giving the worry time to decline.

This is not the same as trying to make yourself so busy that you stop worrying. That's just another version of "stop thinking that" and just as unhelpful in the long run.

Take Your Worries for a Walk

If you have dogs, you generally need to take those dogs for a walk, unless you have room to let them run. There will be times when you don't feel like it—when it's cold and snowy outside, when you're too busy writing a book, or when you have a headache, and you just don't feel like doing it. But if you don't let those dogs poop and pee outdoors, pretty soon they'll do it indoors. That won't do much for your headache or your book! And then when you take those dogs for a walk, they don't always do what you want. Sometimes they race ahead, trying to pull you along. Sometimes they lag behind, and you have to make them follow. Sometimes they try to eat stuff they shouldn't, or bark at your neighbors.

Those dogs are a lot like your worrisome thoughts. Sometimes they demand attention when you really don't feel like giving it, and sometimes they just don't do things the way you wish they would. But life is better with the walks than without them!

You've probably noticed that you tend to worry less when you're busy and more when you're idle. Episodes of chronic worry often fade faster when you're active. So it will be useful to return your attention and energy back to involvement with the external world around you. By this, I don't mean to simply make yourself busy. That's too much like trying to get rid of the thoughts. Not that there's anything terribly wrong with that, getting rid of the thoughts, if it can be done simply and effectively. It's just that trying directly to get rid of the thoughts usually makes them more persistent and plentiful.

So it is with worries. It might seem like there would be a better time to go to a dinner party, but life is a come-as-you-are party, and if you're worried the night of the party, then pack up your worries and bring them with you. Would you be happier without the worries? Yes, but that choice isn't immediately available. Would you be better off lying in bed, alone with your worries? Probably not!

Go on about your business—the worries may leave sooner that way. If they don't, at least you're participating in life while you wait for them to pass.

People often object to the idea of getting involved with a project of any kind, on the grounds that they will be able to do a better job when they're not worried so much. Similarly, they often want to isolate themselves from others, out of a concern that others will notice their distress and be bothered by it.

Both are instances of how our gut instincts of how to handle worry tend to be the opposite of what would actually be helpful. Both suggest that we need, first, to get rid of the worrisome thoughts we're experiencing, and then, afterwards, to get involved with activities outside our skin.

It's more often the other way around. Your involvement with your external world will tend to direct your energy and attention there—and leave less of it "in your head." Moreover, when you interact with the external world, you get more involved with realistic rules of thumb. When you're in your head, by contrast, you can imagine anything. This is why anticipatory worry is almost always worse than anything that actually happens in real life—there are no rules in your head, anything seems possible! In the external world, the rules of reality apply.

Thinking It Over

In this chapter, we looked at an acronym you can use to guide your responses to chronic worry whenever it crops up. The acronym is AHA!

Acknowledge and accept.

Humor *the worrisome thoughts, as you would humor Uncle Argument.*

Activity—resume doing things that are important to you in your "external world" (and take the worries with you if necessary).

You've noticed the worrisome thoughts, and acknowledged them. You've sidestepped the instinct to oppose them and instead cultivated an accepting attitude toward the temporary condition of being worried.

You've responded to the thoughts in some playful ways, perhaps using a song or a poem to play with the content, rather than taking it seriously.

You've gotten back into the external world, and some activity that's meaningful to you. And you allowed the worries to accompany you, if that's what they do.

Treating your worries in this manner—how does it compare to what you usually do?

If it's the opposite of what you usually do, then good! You're on track with the Rule of Opposites.

In chapter 10, we'll consider some regular steps you can build into your daily routine to reduce the amount of chronic worry you experience going forward.

Your Daily Worry Workout

This chapter introduces three daily maintenance tasks you can use to reduce your daily dose of worry and render the worry less disruptive over time. The first one involves regular exposure to worrisome thoughts. The second is a breathing exercise, and the third is a mindfulness meditation.

Use these as you would use a daily vitamin. They're not antibiotics, or some other medication you take to relieve a specific ailment or symptom. They're something you do on a regular basis, not to achieve some immediate, specific goal, but for their overall contribution to your health and wellness.

If you tried the experiment in chapter 8, you probably discovered that when you deliberately turned your attention to chronic worry, without resistance or distraction, your worry lost some of its emotional impact. My clients generally report that they get more relief from deliberate worry than they ever did from thought stopping.

They're usually surprised by that, because it's so—you guessed it—*counterintuitive*. They thought they'd get more relief from efforts to stop worrying than they would from deliberate worry. But it turns out that the opposite is usually true. You'll probably find yourself encountering this realization time and again, as you work with the pattern of chronic worry. The Rule of Opposites is one of the best guides you have!

Chapter 9 offered a variety of quick ways to respond, on the fly, when you find yourself engaged in unwanted chronic worry. They all incorporated the Rule of Opposites, and some of them might have seemed silly. This isn't because I'm silly, or because I think you're silly. It's because so much of the content of chronic worry is silly, and when you take that content at face value, you get fooled into fighting worry in ways that make it worse rather than better. Those responses are all good ways around this problem. I hope you've sampled them, and picked a couple that you can use when the need arises.

Responding to Intermittent Worry

Let's suppose you're the manager of a medium-sized department at your workplace. You have your own work to do, and you have to supervise the work of a group of employees as well. You've tried several different ways to find the right balance between communicating with your staff and getting your own work done.

You tried leaving your door open all the time, so that staff could drop in to see you whenever they want. This encouraged them to stay in touch with you, and to advise you of situations that needed your attention, but it also encouraged a steady stream of staffers dropping by to chat, complain, and score brownie points with you, preventing you from getting your own work done.

Then you tried keeping your door closed, to discourage all but the most determined of staffers. However, this led staffers to increasingly hang around outside your office, sitting around idly, and making noise, while hoping to have a chance to catch your eye. The bolder ones would even knock on your door, or slip notes underneath it. Everyone's productivity, yours and theirs, suffered as a result.

In that case, you might try a third method—setting a schedule for when staffers can drop in and see you, and also for when they should leave you alone unless they smell smoke. You might keep your door closed for much of the day, so you could do your work, and have it open at scheduled times each day, so your staff could see you when they need to. That's the method I want to suggest to you for establishing a better relationship with chronic worry—schedule regular appointments for it.

You'd probably prefer being completely free of worry, but you also probably know by now that avoiding and opposing just gives it more energy. Worry appointments are more likely to help you. They're designed for those persistent, unwelcome worries which are not of any use to you—chronic "what if" worries, which don't point out problems you need to solve, but simply nag and bother you. They build on a feature of worry that you probably noticed when you did the experiment in chapter 8—turning yourself over to worrisome thoughts without resistance usually relieves them of their power.

Set Up Appointments for Worrying

This is time you set aside exclusively for worry. This idea may seem strange to you, because it runs counter to our usual instincts. But that's often how it seems when you "fight fire with fire."

"Fight fire with fire" isn't just a metaphor. It's a technique used to control forest fires. It involves deliberately burning all the flammable material that would otherwise fuel the fire in its spread. When the forest fire arrives at the burned-out part, it falters because it has no fuel left to keep it burning.

Resistance is the fuel by which chronic worry spreads.

During a worry appointment, which will last about ten minutes, you'll engage in pure worry. Devote your full attention to worrying, and nothing else. Don't engage in other activities, like driving, showering, eating, cleaning, texting, listening to music, riding on a train, and so on. Spend the full ten minutes worrying about whatever items you usually worry about. Make a list of your worries ahead of time, so you have an agenda, or use the list you developed in chapter 9. And don't try to solve problems, reassure yourself, minimize problems, relax, clear your mind, reason with yourself, or take any other steps to stop worrying. Simply worry, which means reciting, repeatedly, lots of "what if" questions about unpleasant possibilities.

This will probably seem strange and awkward at first. However, if you're reading this book, you'll likely have lots of experience with worrying. Here's a chance to use that experience for your benefit!

Schedule these times in advance, two a day, and write them into your schedule. Pick times when you have privacy and don't have to answer the phone or the doorbell, talk to others, look after the dog or the kids, and so on. It's usually best to avoid the following times: first thing in the morning on waking, last thing at night, or right after meals.

Watching Yourself Worry

One more detail: worry out loud, in front of a mirror.

This is perhaps the most peculiar part, I know, but don't skip it. It's important!

The advantage of doing the worrying this way is that it helps you be a better *observer* of your worry. Most worry is subliminal. It occurs when we're multitasking. We worry while driving, attending lectures, showering, eating, watching television, or doing some routine work that doesn't demand much attention. And since we rarely give worry our full attention, it's easy for it to continue endlessly.

Because worry comes in the form of our own subliminal thoughts, it has more power to influence us. And we all tend to assume that *If it's my thought, there must be something to it.* We tend not to notice that we can think all kinds of nonsense, that thoughts are often only anxiety symptoms, nothing more.

When you worry out loud, you don't just say the worries, you hear them. When you worry in front of a mirror, you see yourself doing the worrying. You're not just worrying in the back of your mind. You're hearing, and watching, yourself as you worry. The worry is no longer subliminal, and this will probably help you get a better perspective on it.

Worry appointments are deliberately structured this way to convert worry from a multitasking activity to a unitary one, in which you only do one thing—worry—and you do it with the fullest awareness and attention possible.

Why Would Anyone Do This?

Watching yourself worry sounds, on the surface, like a bizarre, unwelcome exercise. You'd need a pretty good reason to do worry appointments.

And there is one! There's usually a benefit that comes during the rest of the day, when you're not engaged in a worry appointment. If you find yourself worrying when you're off "worry duty," you can give yourself the following choice: You can either

a) take ten minutes now to worry very deliberately about this issue, or

b) postpone it to your next worry appointment.

The payoff. The immediate benefit is the ability to postpone worry. Many of my clients find that this enables them to sweep large portions of their day relatively clear of worry. However, it only works if you actually do the worry periods as prescribed. If you try to postpone worries, knowing that you probably won't actually show up for the worry appointments, the postponing probably won't work for you. So don't try to fool yourself!

The postponing alone, the reduction in worry during the rest of your day, would probably be sufficient reason by itself to justify doing worry appointments. But there's more! The regular use of worry appointments will also be a big help in changing your automatic responses to chronic worry, and help you take the content of the worrisome thoughts less seriously.

Taking action about worry is usually much more helpful than thinking about it, reasoning with it, or trying to change the thoughts "in your head." Worry appointments are a good example of this. How about trying it now? Take ten minutes and do the exercise as I describe it above, and then come back to finish this chapter. Or, if this isn't a convenient time for a worry appointment, maybe mark this page in the book, do a worry appointment at a convenient time and location later today, and then return to this page. I encourage you to try it. Doing is better than thinking!

Common Reactions to Worry Appointments

I've worked with a lot of clients who came to see me for help with chronic worry, and I've asked most of them to use worry appointments. I've heard a lot of comments and reactions from people who tried them, and it's usually not the reactions you might expect. When I first started offering this technique, I half expected to get angry feedback that I was an idiot and that they weren't ever coming back! But that's not at all what's happened.

Perhaps the most common reaction clients have is that they tell me, "Boy, it's really hard to fill the ten minutes!" This confused me at first, because these were people who worried a lot, and their days were often filled with worry. So how could it be hard to fill ten minutes? I wondered if it was just an excuse to avoid doing the appointments.

However, as I explored this further with clients, here's what I discovered. They would start the worry appointment and fill a minute or two, and then not have any new worries to add. Normally, when they worried in a subliminal manner, they just kept repeating the worries again and again, and that's what enabled them to worry for such long periods of time. They kept repeating themselves!

But when they did a worry appointment, they assumed they needed to have ten minutes of *fresh* material, without repeating themselves. And they couldn't think of that many worries!

This points to a very important aspect of chronic worry. Although people often have the experience of worrying for long periods of time throughout the day, there are actually very few new worries surfacing during that time. It's almost all repetition of the same minute or two of worrisome thoughts. That's what made it seem hard to fill the ten minutes!

So, when you do worry appointments, don't be concerned with having new, fresh worries each time. During the worry appointments, do what you do when you're worrying spontaneously—just keep repeating the same old worries. If you have two minutes of worry material, repeat that five times, and there's your ten minutes!

If you prefer, you can make up some new ones. Or I can lend you some of mine! The content of the worries during your worry appointment isn't any more important than it is when you're worrying the old-fashioned way. The important thing is simply to fill the ten minutes with the activity of worrying.

Another reaction I often hear goes like this: "I'm not sure I'm getting the same quality in my worries," or "It feels like I'm missing something when I worry this way." When clients tell me this, I usually say something like, "Well, do the best you can!" Of course, I'm kidding when I say that, and we discuss it further. This reaction usually indicates that this person has some beliefs about worry. Without consciously thinking it through, this person has developed some ideas about the "value" of worry, and to worry this way does imply a challenge to those ideas.

These beliefs include such ideas as *It helps to expect the worst* and *Worry shows I care.* A person who harbors the belief that worry somehow can have a beneficial effect on the future will naturally feel nervous when they first start to worry less, for fear that they're not properly taking care of the future by worrying. I'll take a look at these beliefs in chapter 11.

The use of worry appointments takes some commitment. I suggest you try it several times in the next few days. If it seems to work for you the way I describe in this chapter, then I encourage you to do regular appointments for the next two weeks. Review it again after two weeks and make a decision then about continuing or discontinuing.

I find that most people want to discontinue using the appointments a little sooner than I would recommend, but that's all right. If, as often happens, they find that the chronic worry habit starts to creep in again after discontinuing, they can always resume, and stay with it for a longer time. It's probably inconvenient and annoying to do regular worry appointments, and that's why people are so often motivated to stop, even when they see the benefits. I think most people get a more permanent long-term improvement by staying with the worry appointments for months, rather than weeks.

A good way to commit to this is to keep a brief journal, listing your scheduled worry appointments and making notes of your reactions to the appointment after you complete each one.

Breathing and Worry

Breathing is very often affected by worry and anxiety. We see this most dramatically when a person has a panic attack and feels like he is suffocating for lack of air. He's not—no one suffocates from panic—but he *is* experiencing uncomfortable breathing, which tricks him into thinking some catastrophe is about to occur. People with chronic worry often experience a less dramatic but very bothersome discomfort with their breathing as well. This can include such symptoms as feeling light-headed and dizzy, numbness and tingling in the extremities, difficulty getting a full breath, tension and heaviness, thoughts of passing out, and increased heart rate.

These symptoms aren't at all dangerous but can grab your attention in ways that make it more difficult to respond to the worry. For this reason, I often find it helpful for people to learn a good breathing exercise. The point of the breathing exercise is not to control your breathing but to make it sufficiently comfortable that you can return your focus to what's more important—responding to chronic worry.

You may have already tried deep breathing and not had much success. The reason for that is that most descriptions of deep breathing are incomplete. You've probably been told, and you've probably also read it as well, that what you need to do is "Take a deep breath." If you're like most people, that advice hasn't helped you much. It's good advice, but it's incomplete. It doesn't tell you *how* to take a deep breath. A good breathing exercise should tell you *how* to take a deep breath, and that's what I'm going to do. Here's the key: When you feel like you can't catch your breath, it's because you forgot to do something. *You forgot to exhale.*

That's right. Before you can take a deep breath, you have to give one away. Why? Because, when you've been breathing in a short, shallow manner (from your chest), if you try to quickly switch to a deep inhale, it's very hard to do. You're very likely to simply take a more labored, shallow breath from your chest. That will give you all the air you need, but it won't feel good.

Go ahead, try that now and see what I mean. Put one hand on your chest, the other on your belly. Use your hands to notice what muscles you're using to breathe. Breathe very shallowly from your chest a few times, then try to take a deep breath. I think you'll find that when you inhale, you continue to use your chest muscles rather than your diaphragm or belly. Deep breathing, by contrast, comes from your belly.

When you breathe in this shallow manner, you get all the air you need to live, but you can also get other physical symptoms which add to your discomfort. You might get chest pain or heaviness, because you've tightened the muscles of your chest to an uncomfortable degree. You might feel lightheaded or dizzy, because shallow breathing can produce the same sensations as hyperventilation. You might also get a more rapid heartbeat, and maybe numbness or tingling in the extremities as well.

All from breathing short and shallow!

Breathing is actually a sideshow in dealing with chronic worry. The most important response to chronic worry is to use the techniques in this book to develop a different relationship with worry. However, belly breathing can help in managing the

physical symptoms of anxiety while you learn how to relate differently to worry. Use it for periodic comfort when you feel the
need (but don't turn it into another method of opposing and
resisting worry).

Belly Breathing Exercise

1. Place one hand on your belt line, and the other on your
   chest, right over the breastbone. You can use your hands as
   a simple biofeedback device. Your hands will tell you what
   part of your body, and what muscles, you are using to
   breathe.

2. Open your mouth and gently sigh, as if someone had just
   told you something really annoying. As you do, let your
   shoulders and the muscles of your upper body relax, down,
   with the exhale. The point of the sigh is not to completely
   empty your lungs. It's just to relax the muscles of your upper
   body.

3. Close your mouth and pause for a few seconds.

4. Keep your mouth closed and inhale *slowly* through your
   nose by pushing your stomach out. The movement of your
   stomach precedes the inhalation by just the tiniest fraction
   of a second, because it's this motion which is pulling the air
   in. When you've inhaled as much air as you can comfortably (without throwing your upper body into it), just stop.
   You're finished with that inhale.

5. Pause. How long? You decide. I'm not going to give you a
   specific count, because everybody counts at a different rate,
   and everybody has different size lungs. Pause briefly for
   whatever time feels comfortable. However, be aware that

when you breathe this way, you are taking larger breaths than you're used to. For this reason, it's necessary to *breathe more slowly than you're used to*. If you breathe at the same rate you use with your small, shallow breaths, you will probably feel a little lightheaded from overbreathing, and it might make you yawn. Neither is harmful. They're just signals to slow down. Follow them!

6. Open your mouth. Exhale through your mouth by pulling your belly in.

7. Pause.

8. Continue to repeat steps 4 to 7.

Give it a try now. Go ahead and practice the breathing exercise for a few minutes.

Let your hands be your guide. They will tell you if you're doing this correctly or not. Where is the muscular movement of the breathing? You want it to occur at your stomach; your upper body should be relatively still. If you feel movement in your chest, or notice your head and shoulders moving upwards, start again at step 1, and practice getting the motion down to your stomach.

This might feel awkward and difficult the first few times, because breathing in the short, shallow way is such an old habit for people who struggle with anxiety. Don't let that bother you. It just means you need persistent, patient practice. Breathing style is a habit, and the best way to retrain a habit is lots and lots of repetition of the new habit.

This isn't really something new for you. You used to breathe this way all the time, certainly when you were an infant and young child. In fact, if you want to see some world-class belly breathers, visit the newborns in any maternity ward. They don't breathe with their chests at all—just their tummies, which expand outward when they inhale, and contract inwards when they exhale. Infants don't do chest breathing!

Having Trouble? Tips to Help Learn Belly Breathing

- If you have trouble redirecting your breathing from chest to stomach, practice isolating your stomach muscles first. Interlace your fingers across your stomach, and practice pushing your stomach out, then in, without breathing. As you get good at that, begin to pair it with your breathing.

- Use a variety of postures. When you're sitting down, you may find that leaning back in the chair or leaning forward with your forearms on your thighs makes it a little easier than sitting up perfectly straight.

- Lie on your back. You can put a heavy book or other object on your chest to make it easier to focus on using your stomach muscles.

- Lie on your front, with a pillow beneath your stomach, and pressing your stomach against the pillow.

- Practice in front of a full-length mirror, to see what you are doing.

- If you are unable to breathe comfortably through your nose, due to allergies or any other reason, use your mouth instead. You will need to inhale even more slowly this way, in order to avoid gulping your air.

You'll know you've mastered this technique once your breathing feels more relaxing and soothing.

Build the Habit

How often should you practice deep breathing? As often as possible, in sessions of one minute or so, for two weeks.

When it's time to practice, the first thing to do is notice how you've been breathing. Then sigh, and switch to belly breathing for about one minute, as you continue doing whatever you were doing before you started. Don't interrupt your activity. You want good breathing to be portable!

You'll probably do best if you have a system for reminding yourself to practice. Here are some systems you might use:

- Do the deep breathing every hour, at the top of the hour, during your waking day.

- Use ordinary, frequent sounds or occurrences in your daily life as signals to do the breathing. For example, you can do the breathing each time:

  - the dog barks

  - a car horn honks

  - a phone rings

  - someone walks by your office

  - your child drops the sippy cup

  - you receive a text or tweet

- Place stickers or Post-it notes throughout your home, office, or wherever, to remind you.

- Tie a string around your finger.

- Wear your watch on the opposite hand, and practice each time you notice it.

- Set your iPod, wristwatch, or phone to ring periodically.

Do this for two weeks, and you'll be well on your way to changing your breathing for the better!

How Much Is Enough?

People often want to know if they have to breathe this way all the time.

The answer is no.

Just focus on mastering the technique through regular, brief practice. Add it to your list of automatic responses to worry. Use worry appointments, and mindfulness meditation, on a daily basis. And use the belly breathing whenever you feel the need. Over time, I think you'll find that you use this kind of breathing more and more as you make it your new habit. But you can let that happen naturally just by following the suggestions above.

It's Not a Silver Bullet!

Some psychologists and health care professionals believe that professionals such as myself shouldn't teach our clients belly breathing, because people may come to think of the breathing technique as a silver bullet, a lifesaver, and use it the same way they might use any other anti-worry technique.

They have a point.

Still, I find it useful to show this technique to most of my anxious clients because they often have a bad breathing technique, one that creates more anxious physical symptoms. These physical symptoms give rise to more worries and interfere with your ability to handle the anxiety. But keep this point in mind: Belly breathing is best used to help you work with the worry without getting so focused on unrealistic fears of asphyxiation and other physical concerns. Belly breathing will not protect you from physical threats because shallow breathing doesn't actually cause physical calamities.

Mindfulness Meditation

People who aren't accustomed to meditation often think it involves a state of inner peace in which the mind is silent, without all the intrusive thoughts that can interrupt our inner calm. They may occasionally try meditation and feel discouraged when they don't attain this state of inner quiet and calm.

This isn't really what meditation is about, at least for most of us. A monk in a monastery, who devotes large amounts of daily time to meditation, may well obtain significant periods of inner peace and quiet. However, most of us will find that intrusive thoughts initially come to the fore when we set out to meditate and have a quiet mind. So meditation actually consists of noticing, and passively observing, all the thoughts that get in the way when we sit down to have inner peace.

This is particularly the case with mindfulness meditation. It's a process of passively observing thoughts as they come and go while you focus on something basic like your breathing. Don't try to engage in any discussion with your thoughts, nor try to silence or remove them in any manner. Simply observe them.

I attended a meditation workshop years ago at a conference. The workshop was held in a room adjacent to another workshop led by a speaker with a booming voice. I could hear everything this other speaker said as I tried to follow the meditation instructions. I focused on my breath, but kept having thoughts about what a stupid arrangement this was, and those thoughts disrupted my meditation. I had thoughts about the content of what the other speaker (whom I knew personally) was saying and I got irritated with him. I got irritated with the leader of my workshop for asking us to meditate in such noisy circumstances, and irritated with the conference sponsors for selecting such inadequate facilities. I probably looked passive and contemplative, as I sat there, eyes closed, but inside I had a raging storm of thoughts as I struggled to meditate while my unhappy, complaining thoughts grew louder and more numerous. Having thoroughly criticized the workshop, the conference, the sponsors, and the facility, my thoughts moved on to criticize myself, asking, *What is wrong with you that you can't just sit here and relax?* I was actually entertaining thoughts of getting up and walking out when I noticed another thought drift across my mental horizon: *That's just the way you are.* That simple thought allowed me to notice and accept my limitations, and I got back to the task of observing my thoughts. That's meditation.

In this section is a simple practice of mindfulness meditation that can be of help in changing your relationship with chronic worry. (I also offer a recorded version on the website for this book: http://www.newharbinger.com/33186.) Some readers may like it well enough that they are motivated to look more deeply into meditation, to take some instruction and become further involved with meditation as a part of life. That would be great! There's a lot of value to meditation. For others, this simple starter dose of meditation might be all you need.

Want to try it?

Do you immediately find, in your mind, reasons to postpone this, or to "think about it" before you experiment with it? This is a common occurrence. You can notice that thought for what it is, a thought, without becoming engaged with the apparent content of the thought. In other words, you can have the thought about waiting for a better time or opportunity to meditate, and simply do the experiment now anyway. Nobody says you have to do an excellent job of it, or pick the best time to do it. It's just an experiment.

What's that you say? You really have a good reason to wait? You're on a train, or sitting in a waiting room waiting for a doctor? You have a headache, and could probably do a better job some other time? You're too restless...or too tired...or too hungry? Those are excellent thoughts! You can have those thoughts, and you can also do the experiment. If you're willing, go ahead and practice "yes, and," rather than "yes, but."

Here's the exercise:

1. Sit quietly and comfortably somewhere you can be relatively free of interruption for five to ten minutes.

2. Take a minute or two to slow down, sit comfortably erect, and turn your attention to your own thoughts and sensations. It probably helps to close your eyes if you want.

3. Lightly focus your attention on your breathing. Let your attention follow it, as you inhale and exhale. Notice the flow of air as it passes through your nose, your throat, and your lungs. Notice the sensation of your belly as it expands and contracts. Let your attention focus more and more closely on these sensations, as you withdraw your attention from the sights and sounds of the room you occupy. If you don't want to use your breath as a focus, the sound of a fan or something similar will suffice.

4. You may experience some brief moments of quiet, and you can focus, lightly, on that experience. Sooner or later, probably sooner, any inner quiet will get interrupted by automatic thoughts. Simply notice those thoughts, without becoming strongly involved in judging them. Simply allow

your attention to passively return to your focus when you are interrupted or distracted by thoughts. For most people, meditation is not the achievement of internal quiet. *It's noticing the interrupting thoughts that come to mind when you seek internal quiet.*

5. The interrupting thoughts may clamor for your attention. Notice the forms they take to grab your attention. The thoughts may embody not just worry but also judgments, criticisms, anger, regrets, and more.

6. Notice the thoughts the way you might notice drops of rain or snow falling onto your windshield, briefly holding your attention until they're swept away by the windshield wipers and replaced by more raindrops or snowflakes. You don't need to become deeply involved with each snowflake to become aware that there is plenty of snow, and you don't need to become deeply involved with each thought to notice that there is plenty of worry, judgment, criticism, and more in your thoughts as they come and go. Notice their coming and going.

There, you've meditated!

What's that you say? You don't feel any calmer? That's okay. If you had just done your first set of abdominal crunches, your stomach wouldn't be any harder now either. However, with time and repetition, you will probably notice some gradual changes.

You're annoyed at how the thoughts interrupted your effort to feel calm? That's okay. Remember, meditation is about passively observing the thoughts as they rise up to interrupt the quiet. As you experience reactions of annoyance, or an urge to resist, you can notice those thoughts as well.

You don't feel like you did anything? That's okay. This is a brief introduction to experiencing the absence of effort, and the simple observation of thoughts as thoughts, rather than important messages or warnings. It's likely to feel like "doing nothing" if you're in the habit of responding strongly to your automatic thoughts.

You fell asleep? Well, that's a problem. You can't meditate while you're sleeping. Maybe you need to experiment with a different chair, one that's less conducive to sleep, or perhaps you can sit on the floor, with your back against the wall.

Get in the Habit

How about getting some regular experience with this process? Once a day, set aside five to ten minutes for meditation. Just take that time to go through the steps. You might find yourself having thoughts about how well, or poorly, you did the exercise, and you can notice those thoughts as you go, just like all the others. Just show up, go through the steps, and give the habit a chance to develop. After you become more accustomed to the practice, increase your daily time to ten to twenty minutes.

Our days are often filled with activities that we have to *make* happen, and it's easy to forget that there are also activities that we just *allow* to happen. People who experience chronic worry are likely to think that they need to control the thoughts they experience, and make themselves experience the thoughts they want to have, rather than the ones that occur spontaneously. It usually doesn't work so well.

The chief benefit of adding this technique to your daily activities is that it will help you become a better, and more dispassionate, observer of your own thoughts. Over time you will enhance your own ability to observe thoughts without becoming embroiled in the content of the thoughts.

People who struggle with chronic worry are sometimes hesitant to sample meditation because they have thoughts that suggest that maybe they'll just encounter more unpleasant thoughts, and more struggle with those thoughts, when they meditate. My experience is that people generally find the opposite to be true. Experience with meditation usually leads people to be more tolerant and accepting of whatever thoughts they happen to encounter.

It's the Rule of Opposites!

Thinking It Over

This chapter prescribes three activities for daily use that can help to moderate the amount of worry you experience on a daily basis. These can be the basis for a good maintenance program for keeping your relationship with chronic worry more evenhanded.

CHAPTER II

The Worry Parasite

Chronic worry functions like a parasite, increasingly getting the host—that's you!—to spend time and energy on producing and maintaining worry, rather than pursuing the hopes and dreams you have for your own life. This chapter will look at how it does this, and suggest a way out.

But first, I want to tell you the story of a parasitic flatworm, the formal name for which is *Leucochloridium paradoxum*.

Yes, I know, my family wasn't much interested in this story either. But I think once you've read it, you'll have a better appreciation of what's at stake here, and how the worry game is played.

How a Parasite Takes Over a Snail

This parasitic flatworm is a microscopic creature and is often found living inside amber snails. It spends a large portion of its life cycle inside snails, but when it comes time to reproduce and make baby parasites, it can only do this inside the belly of a bird, which is its preferred environment. There it can live off the bird's food and have a secure home in which to lay eggs, which will give rise to new generations of parasites. The eggs it lays return to the ground in bird droppings.

The parasite spends much of its life cycle inside a snail, which crawls around on the ground, under rocks and leaves. So how, you might wonder, does it get inside the belly of a bird?

The amber snail likes to eat bird droppings. When these droppings contain parasitic eggs, baby flatworms hatch inside the snail and begin a nefarious plot of mind control.

The first thing these flatworms do is locate the brain of the snail—and if you've ever had trouble finding a small lost item at home, imagine what a job this is, finding the brain of a snail! But they find the brain, and bring to it a substance, a hormone or a neurotransmitter.

The chemical that the flatworm brings to the snail's brain leads the snail to act differently than before. The snail no longer moves "at a snail's pace" but moves about much more rapidly. All activities which serve the purposes of the parasite are maximized, and all activities that only serve the purpose of the snail are eliminated or greatly reduced. The snail no longer seeks out other snails with which to mate. If focuses exclusively on moving around rapidly and getting food.

But that's not all! Now, under the influence of the flatworms, the snail has a whole new view of life.

The snail has the ability to change its outer color. Normally, the snail favors dull, bland colors, a thousand shades of brown, which blend into its environment and hide it from predators. But now the snail "thinks" to itself, *I've always wanted colored eyestalks!* Its eyestalks blossom into bright colors. And the flatworms find their way to the snail's eyestalks. Normally the snail can retract its eyestalks at will, but the flatworms engorge and fatten the eyestalks to the point where they can't retract. The flatworms hop around in the brilliantly colored eyestalks, making them pulsate and appear to move, looking for all the world like a caterpillar on the move. (Search *Leucochloridium paradoxum* on the Internet if you want to see videos!)

And, under the continuing influence of the flatworms, the snail now thinks, *I've always wanted to sunbathe!* So the snail, which heretofore has always preferred to stay in dark, shady places, now climbs to the top of a tree and basks in the sun, displaying its brilliantly colored, caterpillar-resembling eyestalks.

And the next thing you know, the parasites are inside the belly of a bird! Birds generally don't eat snails, but they're so attracted by the eyestalks that look like caterpillars that they pluck them off for a tasty meal, leaving the snail to grow a new pair. This goes on for the rest of the snail's life. It's become a zombie snail, functioning as a host for more parasites.

The parasite has literally hijacked the self-care agenda of the snail. The snail now acts in ways that further the purposes and interests of the parasitic flatworms, rather than the purposes and interests of the snail.

That's what chronic worry does. Chronic worry literally hijacks your own self-care agenda and makes it serve the maintenance of chronic worry, rather than your plans, dreams, hopes, and aspirations. That's how insidious this is. Your life becomes more about worry and less about your work, your relationships, your fun, your intellect—everything that makes life worthwhile.

How Worry Takes Over Your Life

How does this happen? And how can you roll this process back and regain control of how you spend your time and energy in life?

You probably get a sense of how your life agenda has been hijacked when you recall how much time and energy you spend not just worrying, but also engaging in the anti-worry techniques we looked at in chapter 3. What did you used to do with all the time and energy that now gets tied up in worry and anti-worry? You probably actually *did* more things, things that were important to you in your role as parent, spouse, friend, neighbor, employee, and so on. You had interests, passions, and ambitions that you wanted to follow. And you probably followed them and did things with a lot less mental struggle than you experience now.

It's not that you didn't worry at all. You certainly did, because everybody worries to some extent. But you were probably more likely to go ahead and engage in activities that were important to you. You gave the speech to the PTA or some other public meeting, even though you were nervous about public speaking; you went on vacation to an unfamiliar place, even though you had worries about getting lost or feeling out of place; you sold your home and moved elsewhere, even though you had doubts if it was the right thing to do; you had an annual physical, even though you were a little nervous it would find something bad; you applied for a new job, even though you were nervous about interviewing and weren't sure if it was the right time for a job change, and so on.

The Parasitic Effects of Worrying

When you get caught up in chronic worry, it doesn't just disturb your peace of mind. Chronic worry leads to systematic changes in the way you think and behave, just as the parasitic flatworm changes the behavior of the snail. And these changes don't further your own values and aspirations; they further the maintenance of the worry, just as the changes in snail behavior favor the parasite's interests, rather than the snail's.

Chronic worry redirects much of your time, attention, and energy to worry rather than life. It leads you to spend more and more time "in your head," in your internal world, trying to get your thoughts arranged the way you think they should be, always struggling and fussing with worry rather than getting out into your external world and living, doing whatever it takes to be the good parent, good friend, good employee, good neighbor, or good whoever you always wanted to be. It leads you to invest your time and energy in worry, and struggles with worry, rather than in being the person you wanted to be and living the life you hoped for.

This Invasion Began with Certain Beliefs

How does chronic worry hijack your agenda? The hijacking of the snail starts when it ingests the parasitic eggs. Your hijacking started when you adopted and developed certain types of beliefs about worry. Over time, maybe all the way back in early childhood, you developed some beliefs about worry. These are typically beliefs that you rarely notice or reflect upon, beliefs which have a strong influence on how you think and how you act. Much of their power comes from the fact that you rarely notice or reflect upon the thoughts, and so they exert a powerful subliminal influence, much like propaganda.

These beliefs all have an ironic aspect, because they all consider worry to have value. It probably sounds silly to say that, because doesn't everyone recognize that worry is a useless activity? Isn't that why people who struggle with chronic worry want to overcome it, because they realize it's a useless diversion of their time and energy? But it's not as simple as that. If you consider closely how you react to worry, I think you will find evidence that whatever you may say or think about worry being nonsensical and pointless, you actually do behave, some of the time, as if worry has some important value and power all by itself.

People don't often talk about these beliefs with others, and often don't directly think about the beliefs. Most people don't recommend worry to others, and you probably don't either. At first glance, when you look at these beliefs below, you might be likely to dismiss them as having nothing to do with you. But give each one a little consideration.

It helps if I expect the worst.

I've talked with so many people who subscribe to this idea. It seems to them that, if they expect the worst, they won't ever be surprised or experience an overwhelming feeling about some sudden bad event. For them, worry is a kind of dress rehearsal for bad events that might happen in the future. They rehearse and study their lines, the scene, and their likely reactions, and feel dread now, somehow thinking this will protect them from feeling really bad someday, as though worry were a vaccine against feeling overwhelmed in the future.

People who are influenced by this belief don't like to feel optimistic. They're suspicious of optimism because they think the universe, or God, will "even things out" by giving them something bad because they're feeling optimistic. This has a superstitious aspect to it, as when people "knock on wood" because they just said something optimistic, and they hope to prevent that statement from backfiring on them.

They may also think that God, or the universe, is likely to give them something good when they feel pessimistic. They often think of "expecting the worst" as a kind of preparation for bad events, a form of "paying your dues."

Questions to Consider

Have you ever felt a little nervous because you voiced an optimistic prediction, or had an optimistic thought?

Have you ever felt like you should do something to "undo" that thought, some version of "knock on wood"?

Have you ever experienced difficult events without emotional upset, like the death of a parent or the loss of a job, because you did enough worrying about it ahead of time?

Have you experienced difficult events you did not anticipate? Were you able to manage the emotional upset despite your lack of worry preparation?

Have you worried significantly about events that never occurred? (Did you just think *Not yet, they haven't?*) What percentage of the things you worry about have actually happened?

Want to Do an Experiment?

Try holding some optimistic thoughts to see if the simple act of holding positive thoughts makes you a little nervous.

My kids will be happy and healthy every day this week, without any problems.

I know I'm in excellent health and won't contract any diseases.

All my friends and relatives will be safe from harm this week.

Hold these thoughts in mind for a couple of minutes, and see how you feel about them. If holding these thoughts makes you a little uncomfortable, it's probably because you do tend to believe, at some level, that *It helps if I expect the worst.*

My worry can influence future events.

When you're under the influence of this belief, you tend to act as if the simple act of worrying can change the future, that it might prevent bad events from happening that would have otherwise happened. I'm not referring here to situations in which your thoughts lead you to take action, and those actions influence the future. Here I mean that people treat worry itself as something that can affect the future.

This belief can make worry seem like a double-edged sword. On the one hand, if you worry about the "right" things, maybe the worry will prevent bad things from happening. On the other, if you fail to worry about them, maybe this will cause bad things to happen. How can you ever be sure which are the right things to worry about? This idea sure makes worry seem important!

Now, if this idea were really true, we wouldn't need to spend trillions on the military—we could just organize our civilians into worrying about war. We'd draft worriers, rather than warriors! But then we'd have to worry about whether we were preventing war or causing it.

Unlikely as it seems, many people subscribe to this idea, sometimes in a superstitious way. They may actually feel nervous when they notice that they've been worrying less, as if somehow they stopped paying their dues, and they need to get that payment in the mail right away.

Questions to Consider

Have you ever noticed that you hadn't been worrying about a topic that you had been worrying about a great deal?

Did it make you feel a little nervous?

Did you feel a little irresponsible, like you hadn't been doing your job?

Did you think you should resume worrying about it? Did you resume worrying about it?

If something bad happens and I hadn't worried about it, I'll feel guilty.

This belief leads you to treat worry as a duty, or maybe even a beneficial activity. If you shirk your duty, bad things will happen and they'll be your fault.

It's certainly true that if there's something you're supposed to *do* (say, water your plants) and you fail to do it (and they die), then that's your fault. But there's a big difference between worrying and doing.

Questions to Consider

Has this idea ever led you to worry?

Have you ever felt guilty for not worrying about something that actually happened?

Did you apologize to anyone who was harmed or bothered by the event? Did you make amends?

Were you able to forgive yourself?

Worry shows I care.

This is a surprisingly widespread belief. It shows how we often fail to recognize the important distinction between thoughts and action.

If you have children, you probably want to be a caring parent, and also to be seen as a caring parent by your family and friends. The best way, probably the only way, to judge how much parents care for their children is to look at their actions. Do they attempt to fill the child's needs, physical and emotional? Do they make an effort to balance assisting the child and fostering independence? Do they work at the very difficult task of communicating with the child through the various developmental stages of childhood?

Caring is demonstrated by doing. Yet in our culture, we do tend to attribute some positive characteristics to worry. It's so common for people to reflexively, automatically, think that caring is somehow demonstrated by worrying.

Questions to Consider

If you were told that a neighbor never worries about his kids, would you think that was a good thing or a bad thing?

Would you like to be known as someone who doesn't worry about your kids?

If your significant other said to you, "I don't think you ever worry about me," would you take it as a complaint or a compliment?

Thoughts are always important.

It's a very basic human frailty to assume that thoughts are always important, and especially that one's own thoughts are particularly wise and important. It's a kind of vanity. Our brain produces thoughts, and if we want to evaluate our thoughts, we have to go back to the organ that produced them in the first place. No wonder we often think they're more important than they are!

If you've ever had a song stuck in your head, you've had the experience of noticing that some thoughts, like song lyrics, get very stuck in your mind, despite their lack of importance.

When you're anticipating some kind of potentially difficult encounter with another person—say, you're going to ask for a raise, or talk to a neighbor about his noisy dog—you might repeatedly find thoughts playing in your head as you imagine how the conversation will go.

How often do those thoughts turn out to be accurate, and how often does the encounter go the way you anticipated?

I am responsible for my thoughts.

If you could pick and choose what thoughts you have, and what thoughts you don't have, there might be something to this idea. Certainly it would be good to use your powers of mind control wisely, if you had such powers, and if your thoughts affected those you love.

Do your thoughts affect the people around you?

Do you control your thoughts?

Let's see. Can you now hold in mind a flag without any red, white, or blue colors in it?

I think you'll find, when you consider these questions, that your thoughts have no influence on anyone else, unless you choose to share them, and even then the effect of sharing your thoughts with others is unpredictable.

I think you'll also find that, while you can apply your thoughts to a problem like a crossword puzzle or a tax calculation, you also have thoughts that occur to you spontaneously, even when you wish they wouldn't.

What Beliefs Do You Hold About Your Thoughts?

Make a list of the worry beliefs you hold. This will give you the opportunity to decide how you want to relate to these beliefs. Do you want to continue to act in accordance with these beliefs? Do you want to play with them? What would the Rule of Opposites suggest about responding to these beliefs?

Thinking It Over

Chronic worry can slowly, almost invisibly, infiltrate your beliefs and your life in ways that hijack your hopes and dreams for your life and turn you into an agent of worry rather than a person who lives the life he wants. Identifying these beliefs, and applying the Rule of Opposites, can do for you what killing off the parasites would do for the amber snail.

Breaking the Secrecy Trap

When you have an ongoing struggle with chronic worry, you probably often feel frustrated by the way in which friends and loved ones "just don't get it" about this problem. All too often, they offer simpleminded solutions like "Don't worry so much," or even imply that it's your fault. They may be genuinely confused about how to be helpful, sometimes saying what they think you want to hear in an effort to help you calm down, other times refusing to discuss the problem at all. This chapter suggests ways you can get the helpful support you may need to change your relationship with worry for the better.

Are You Keeping Your Worries to Yourself?

Who knows about the problem you have with chronic worry? What do they know about it?

If you're like most people with chronic worry, you probably haven't told many people, for a variety of reasons. Maybe you're embarrassed and fear that others will lose respect for you if they know about your trouble with worry. Maybe you don't want to cause others to worry about you. Maybe you're afraid that if you talk about it, you'll make it worse somehow, that just acknowledging it out loud might make it a bigger problem; or that if others know about your worry, they'll keep asking if you're worried in ways that continually rekindle your worry.

We'll come back to those thoughts later in this chapter. First, I want to direct your attention to what the urge for secrecy reveals about worry. Most people who struggle with worry—or any kind of anxiety, for that matter—tend to keep it secret. What does it tell me about a problem if I'm motivated to keep it a secret? What kinds of problems are we motivated to keep secret?

Give that a little thought while I tell you about someone who kept his worry a secret. Allan (not his real name) had a persistent worry about contamination by some unhealthy substance. His worry wasn't that he would become contaminated, or that he would carelessly cause contamination. His worry was that he might be present when some kind of contamination posed a danger to people, and that he would either fail to notice it or, if he did notice, that he wouldn't take effective action to protect others. Then, he feared, he would carry the guilt of failing to protect those who were subsequently harmed by the contamination.

It seemed a little far-fetched, even to him, but he could never really "be sure"; at the same time, he felt the possibility of people being harmed required that he be sure whenever possible. One evening he was at a party and noticed what he took to be a contaminated Styrofoam cup adjacent to the punch bowl. He described to me how he worked his way across the room and stood in front of the punch bowl so that no one could see what he was doing. Behind his back, he counted down through the stack of cups to the one he suspected was contaminated, and removed it. He surreptitiously crushed the cup in his hand and placed it in his pocket for safe disposal later.

When Allan finished telling me this story, I acknowledged his good intentions in seeking to protect people from the contaminated cup. I asked him why he hadn't simply walked over to the punch bowl, told everyone about the contaminated cup, and removed it while they watched.

Allan laughed, and said, "That would have been really embarrassing! There probably wasn't anything wrong with that cup!" *That's* what the urge to keep your worry a secret can tell you about the problem. There's usually something funny about that worry, something that doesn't stand up in the light of day. That's why you're motivated to keep it a secret.

Keeping Secrets

Does that match your experience? Do you find you're motivated to keep your worries a secret because there's something odd about their content, something that doesn't entirely make sense? If that fits for you, then feeling the urge to keep your worry a secret can be a reminder that there's something funny about that worry, that the worry is just another invitation to "pretend…something bad," as we saw when we diagrammed worry sentences in chapter 6.

When you find yourself wanting to hide your worry, it can be a valuable reminder that you're simply nervous. That's why you're worrying, you're nervous, not because you're up against a real problem in the external world.

You'd probably prefer not to notice it at all, but it's actually helpful to notice your nervousness. Noticing that you're feeling nervous can be a good reminder to do your AHA! steps.

Acknowledge and accept.

Humor the worrisome thoughts, as you would humor Uncle Argument.

Activity—resume doing things that are important to you in your "external world" (and take the worries with you if necessary).

Secrecy and Shame

One of the main reasons people keep their worry a secret is that they feel ashamed of how much worrying they do. They fear others would shame and criticize them if they became aware of the worrying. Protection from this anticipated shame and embarrassment. This is the usual main effect people hope to achieve by keeping their worrying problem a secret, preventing shame and embarrassment.

Maybe you achieve that main effect, avoiding shame and embarrassment, although even that usually feels very temporary to most worriers. They're always worried that they could accidentally reveal their worrisome nature at any time, and so rarely get any long-term comfort from the secrecy. But main effects don't tell the entire story.

If you've ever watched any medication commercials on television, you probably also know about side effects. Maybe you've seen a commercial for some medication that's supposed to relieve a problem, like acid reflux or erectile dysfunction. At the bottom of the screen, in tiny print, comes a long list of unpleasant side effects. Sometimes they sound pretty nasty, or dangerous, even worse than the problem the medicine is supposed to relieve. As a consumer, it's up to you to decide if the benefit of the medication exceeds the problem of whatever side effects you might experience.

There are also side effects to hiding your problem with worry. It would be good to consider these side effects in evaluating whether or not secrecy is a helpful strategy for you. Here are some of the side effects.

Imagining the worst. Keeping your worries hidden, even from people who are close to you, deprives you of any feedback you might receive if you shared the information. You're left on your own to guess at what the worry might mean to them, and how other people would view your difficulties. Since worry always exaggerates the negative and makes the unlikely seem quite probable, your guess of how people might respond to your worries is probably exaggerated and overblown in the same way. The chances are excellent that your guess of how people would think about you and your worries is far worse than what they would actually think, and say, if they knew. So you're left imagining the worst, rather than something more realistic.

Feeling like a fraud. I've worked with many people who were chronic worriers. Many of them were quite successful in different areas of their life, with major accomplishments to their credit. However, they could rarely feel good about their successes. They were preoccupied with this thought: *If people knew how much worrying I do, they wouldn't think very highly of me.* They literally thought they were frauds, and this belief was a negative side effect of the secrecy they maintained.

Increased worry. When you have a secret to keep, it naturally increases your worry, because you're often concerned with the possibility of accidentally revealing your secret.

Increased social isolation. Chronic worry naturally interferes with social interaction with others, because it leads people to spend time "in their heads," arguing with their thoughts, rather than interacting with people. People often cancel social engagements when they feel "too worried" to attend a dinner or a party. When this is accompanied by secrecy, it prevents you from accurately explaining your reasons to the other party, who is left guessing why you canceled the planned luncheon, or why you sometimes seem distant. Because others are likely to think that you're just not interested in them, this can damage your social network.

Paradoxical increase in symptoms. Your thoughts don't shape or cause events outside you, in the external world, but they can shape and cause physical and emotional symptoms of anxiety within you. A person who worries a lot about blushing, or sweating, in a social setting—and keeps those fears a secret—is likely to experience more of those symptoms purely because she is trying so hard to not have them. Similarly, a person who worries about his voice cracking during a presentation probably increases the odds of that symptom.

The overall effect of these side effects of secrecy is this: While you may believe that you are fooling people by keeping your worries secret, only one person is really getting fooled, and that's you. The secrecy fools you into believing that you have a terrible, shameful, insoluble problem and that no one would ever like or respect you if they knew about it.

There might be some good reasons to selectively reveal your struggle with worry, at least to a couple of people who seem to have your best interests at heart. While no one likes the prospect of feeling embarrassed, the feeling of it generally passes pretty quickly. The negative side effects of secrecy, on the other hand, can last a lifetime if you never break the secrecy, so you may find significant benefit in ending it.

When I first talk to a worried client about self-disclosure, he usually says something like this: "I don't want to tell anybody about this problem. It's none of their business!"

That's true. Your worries are nobody's business but your own.

The only reason to discuss it with someone is if you think that it might help *your* business, of living, reducing worry, following your aspirations, and so on. It's about your business, not theirs.

So it might be worthwhile to do a little cost–benefit analysis of the effects of keeping your worry pattern a secret—the main effect, and the side effects listed above as well—to help you decide if you want to experiment with a little selective self-disclosure.

If you decide to experiment with self-disclosure, I have some suggestions for you.

Planning Self-Disclosure

Start with a significant other, or someone fairly central in your social network. Pick someone who's clearly in your corner, someone who will be motivated to hear what you're saying, to understand, and be helpful.

Schedule an agreeable time. Don't just work it in at the end of a phone call or other conversation, and don't leave it to chance. Tell him or her there's something you want to discuss, and ask to set up a specific time and place. Do this in person if at all possible. You don't need a lot of time. Probably fifteen to thirty minutes should be plenty, unless you want more. Your friend will be curious what the topic is, but don't get into it until the time comes. You can reassure him or her that you don't want to borrow any money!

Come right to the point. Don't beat around the bush or spend the first few minutes on small talk, sports, or catching up on general news. Get right into the topic, as suggested in this sample.

> *Thanks for setting this time. The thing I want to talk about is an issue I've been having and it weighs on my mind. I worry a lot, and I know everybody worries, but I think it's a bigger deal for me than for most people.*

Here's a typical description of worrying, but it'll be better to insert your own description here.

> *I find myself thinking and worrying a lot, mostly about stuff that never really happens—or if it does, isn't nearly as bad as I expect—but it really occupies my mind and distracts me from other stuff I'd rather be thinking about. It's kind of embarrassing to talk about, but that's the main reason I wanted to tell you about this, I think it makes it worse if I keep it to myself, keep it in my head. I worry about all kinds of stuff, and have trouble letting it go.*
> *So, the biggest ways this causes me trouble is [here* describe briefly a few ways the worry causes you trouble.

This might include getting distracted, having trouble sleeping, and other results of worrying. It should definitely include some of the ways you struggle to control your worry and get rid of it, discussed in chapter 3. If this is a person you ever approach for reassurance, describe that part of worrying].

You're probably wondering why I'm telling you this. Mainly, I'm thinking it might help me to get this off my chest, to get over keeping it a secret, because I think keeping it to myself makes it seem like a bigger problem to me.

But now that I've told you about this, there're a couple of things I'd like for you to do and not do.

And here is the part where you will probably find it helpful to literally educate others, train them, about what is helpful and not helpful in relating to your worry. People's concerns about how their loved ones and friends will overreact, or respond in unhelpful ways, are one of the reasons they keep it a secret. You can't expect that they will automatically know how to be helpful. You'll have to explain it to them.

Guidelines to Give Your Support People

Don't start asking me "How are you doing—are you worrying?" If I want to talk about this some more, I'll bring it up. I'd rather you didn't initiate it.

Generally, it's not a good thing for you to give me reassurance about something I worry about. I'm likely to overthink it and question it, trying so hard to be "sure" that it just causes more trouble, for me and maybe for you as well. I have to get better at handling uncertainty. If you

*do give me reassurance about something, make it realistic.
Don't tell me something will always be okay, in all ways.
Put the usual realistic disclaimers in there, like "As far as
I know" or "Anything can happen, but what's likely to
happen is…," because I know nothing in the future is
sure, and I have to get used to that.*

*If I appear to be asking you for reassurance about something,
I'd like you to point that out—"It sounds like you're asking
me for reassurance, is that really what you want?"—and
give me a chance to change my mind about that.*

*Don't share this information with anyone. If I want someone
else to know, I'll tell them.*

*Don't go out of your way to try to be helpful, or do things
you think will make my life easier. If there's something I
want or need you to do, I'll ask you. Or, if you think you
have a really good idea, ask me about it, but don't do
anything without asking me first.*

Give this a try with someone who's important in your life
and motivated by your best interests. See how it goes and evaluate what the effects are. If you find the results are at least
neutral, or positive, then perhaps this will encourage you to
begin breaking some of the secretive habits you maintain about
your worry with others.

One good way to do this is to notice when you are offering
up an excuse or making up a story to cover up the fact that you
are worried. For instance, you might find yourself declining an
invitation to lunch with a friend at a fancy restaurant because
you anticipate feeling really uncomfortable there. You don't
want to feel "trapped" at a table in the center of such a place as

you try to "get through" the meal. You picture yourself waiting anxiously for your friend to finish coffee and dessert, then trying to tolerate the delays inherent in getting and paying the bill, when you would much rather rush out of there.

If you catch yourself in the act of offering a fake excuse, simply interrupt yourself and pause, then say something like, "No, I take that back. It's just that sometimes I get antsy in a place like that, especially when I have a lot on my mind like I do now, and I get too restless to enjoy myself. How about we just do something quick and easy?"

This has the virtue of maintaining your social connection with this friend and taking care of your needs. And it opens the door a bit for you to acknowledge a bit of worry that you experience, so you can get a realistic reaction from a friend, rather than the blaming, shaming, secretive reaction you experience when you make excuses.

Getting Support From Another Key Person

There's another person in your life from whom you can probably get more support in your effort to reshape your relationship with chronic worry.

It's you.

You might be different from most of the clients I've worked with. But what I notice about people struggling with chronic worry is that they tend to be so self-critical with themselves that it makes their job harder. They condemn themselves for being worried, as if it were literally their fault, some kind of crime, rather than an unfortunate problem they wrestle with.

They tend to be pretty stingy with praising themselves for their efforts, and all too free with the blame and shame.

While they often complain about how their friends and family "don't get it," they regularly think things to themselves that are far more unhelpful than even their worst enemy would say.

It's not because they don't know how to be supportive and compassionate. These are usually people who are very capable of understanding someone else's problems and offering support, or at least a neutral ear, without criticism.

They just don't give themselves this kind of support. When clients come in and share with me some of the critical self-statements they hear in their internal world, it's surprising how persistently negative they are.

They know how to be supportive with others, but don't use this ability with themselves, in their own internal dialogue. Why not?

I think it's because there aren't any witnesses in there! It happens so automatically they often don't even notice the critical thoughts. They just feel the effect, in terms of feeling demoralized.

Does this sound like something you do? Maybe it would be helpful to keep track of your critical internal monologue for a week or so, just to see what it's like. Keep track, on a pad of paper or a digital device, of how often you find yourself saying harsh and blameful things to yourself in the privacy of your internal world. No need to argue with it, just to observe, and maybe to pause and say, "Oh well—there I go again!"

Thinking It Over

What does it mean if you're motivated to keep your worry a secret? It's often a good indication that there's something exaggerated and unrealistic about that worry. That's a helpful reminder, and if you start looking at the urge to secrecy in that light, it will probably help you respond to your worries in more effective ways.

Keeping your worries secret comes at a price, often a significant one, with serious negative effects of the secrecy. Try the suggestions in this chapter for experimenting with self-disclosure, a little at a time, and judge it by its results, not by your anticipatory fears.

Specialized Worries: Sleep and Illness

In this chapter, I'll look at two specific content areas of worry: sleep and health. Actually, the worries are about feared failures in these areas: worries about failing to sleep, or insomnia; and worries about disease when the worrier doesn't seem to have a disease.

These worries often become closely tied with very specific responses, so I'll describe the responses, explain how they make the problem worse, and offer some specific new responses that will help you unravel the problem. You can skip this chapter if you're not bothered by either of these worries. You might still find it useful, though, for the way it describes how people's behaviors change to fit in with the worries.

Worries About Sleep

Jay was going through a stressful time. He had recently accepted a new position, a job he thought of as the chance of a lifetime. He accepted the job even though he had some concerns about juggling the new workload with his role as a new father. Work was actually going well for the first six months.

Then one night he had trouble sleeping. There was no obvious reason, but he woke up around 2 a.m. feeling anxious. His heart was beating faster than usual, and he felt apprehensive. He thought he had experienced an unpleasant dream, but couldn't remember any details. He lay there for a while, trying to get back to sleep without success. He got up to use the bathroom, had a drink of cool water, checked his e-mail, and then returned to bed, hoping for sleep. He got none. He found himself resenting his wife for the peaceful sleep she seemed to be enjoying, and even the sound of her breathing seemed sufficient to keep him awake. Periodically, he'd look at the clock and calculate how much sleep he could get if he fell asleep right away. This aggravated him and made him less sleepy. Finally, around 5 a.m., he drifted off for a little while, but soon awoke to the sound of his son crying.

Jay went to work feeling a little tired, but the day passed without trouble. However, shortly before leaving the office, he found himself having the thought, *I hope I don't have trouble sleeping again tonight.* The thought bothered him. He could feel his heart beat a little faster, and his breathing got short for a few moments. His thoughts turned to the question *What if I can't sleep tonight?* and he envisioned himself mishandling work tasks because he was so sleep deprived.

Driving home, he found himself wondering what he could do to improve his chances for good sleep. He hit upon a few ideas: he'd have a mug of hot chocolate before bed; he'd skip watching his favorite crime show that night, which was sometimes kind of intense, and read something tame instead; and he'd go to bed early.

Jay worried about sleep throughout the evening, as if he were preparing for a physical challenge. He went to bed an hour earlier than usual, but it didn't help him fall asleep earlier. He just lay there, feeling tense. Concerned, he got up and sat in the living room, watching a talk show and hoping to fall asleep. He fell asleep there, waking a couple of hours later with the TV still on and wondered if he should "risk" going back to the bedroom, or stay where he was. He tried going back to bed, but after a few minutes of anxiety there, he returned to the living room and slept until morning.

He felt apprehensive about going to work and had thoughts about not being alert enough to handle his responsibilities. He drank an extra cup of coffee and tried to get some reassurance from his wife. She pointed out, accurately, that he had gone with a lot less sleep during the first few weeks after the baby was born, but that fact didn't really calm him. Before he left the house, Jay reviewed his schedule to see if there were any meetings or other activities he could cancel. He didn't see any, but looking at his schedule reminded him of the end of the day, and he wondered again, *What if I can't sleep tonight?*

Jay "got through" his workday without incident, but felt on edge, and he tried to think of more strategies to get better sleep. He stopped at the gym on the way home for a good workout, hoping to tire himself. He asked his wife to avoid any mention of negative topics, and hoped his son wouldn't wake him early. He had a glass of warm milk that night, having read that chocolate might hamper sleep, and went to bed early, putting a hand towel over his eyes for extra darkness, and ear plugs in his ears for extra quiet. He tried not to think about waking up at 2 a.m. again. It took him longer than usual to fall asleep, but eventually he did.

Then he woke up at 2 a.m. and went downstairs to sleep on the sofa. Over the next few days, he started sleeping on the sofa instead of the bed, because he found it easier to drift into sleep there, watching TV and not focusing on trying to sleep. Whenever he went upstairs to go back to the bedroom, he worried about failing to fall asleep, and failed to fall asleep. He switched out the glass of warm milk for a glass of cold beer for about a week, until his wife persuaded him to go see his doctor. The doctor gave him a prescription for some sleeping tablets. He used those for a week or so, but didn't like how groggy he felt in the morning, and since the doctor had cautioned him that the pills were only for short-term use, he discontinued taking them.

Jay's experience with sleep worry is typical of what many people experience. They have a night of troubled or interrupted sleep, often for no apparent reason. They worry about it repeating. They try to head it off with a variety of tactics. These tactics treat sleep as if it were a struggle or an accomplishment. They actually make sleep more difficult, build worry about sleep. Worry about sleep is often a classic example of the Rule of Opposites. It so often leads people to respond in ways that make sleep more difficult even as they hope and wish for it to come easily.

Sleep: Let it Happen, or Make it Happen?

Let's start with some basics. What do we do to fall asleep?

Sleep is one of those activities that we *allow* to happen, rather than make happen. How do we do that? We create a space that's quiet, comfortable, and dark, with no distractions or features that encourage waking activity. We show up and lie down, prepared to "let go" of daily concerns and activities, and we give that process a little time to occur.

"Trying to sleep" is a contradiction, because sleep is an activity that doesn't respond well to effort. Think of one of your favorite meals. How likely are you, when served this meal, to scrutinize what you do with teeth and tongue? How likely are you to urge yourself to get more flavor and enjoyment from that meal, and judge how well you are doing at getting that flavor and enjoyment? Probably not so likely! Instead, you sit down at an appropriate place, with the appropriate utensils, have your beverage of choice, put the food in your mouth, and allow the experience to unfold. Even though it's the same dish, it's probably a slightly different experience each time, but you don't score it like an Olympic event unless you're a judge on *Iron Chef.*

Many of our daily activities are the type requiring effort, in which effort is rewarded. The more persistently I teach my dog to stay off the sofa, the better she'll behave, at least as far as the sofa's concerned. The more regular effort I put into my workout, the better my physique and muscle tone, and so on.

Sleep isn't like that. The activity of sleep is more like simple relaxation, enjoying the flavor of your food, or having an orgasm. You arrange the right conditions, go through a few simple steps, and enjoy what comes your way. You don't struggle to create the experience because struggle and enjoyment of these activities are mutually exclusive.

Setting Up Your Bedroom for Restful Sleep

What are the right conditions? This is what sleep psychologists call "sleep hygiene." It doesn't mean having clean sheets, although that's always a plus. It means creating a good environment, and routine, that's conducive to sleep. This means reserving your bed and bedroom for sleep, also for sex, but nothing else. This may be a big adjustment for people who are "plugged in" 24/7.

No TV in the bedroom, get it out of there. Turn off your devices—your phone, your notebooks and other devices—and leave them in the living room. If you have to have something in your bedroom to divert you, one book is sufficient.

Take your clock and turn it to face the wall. When people are having trouble sleeping, they often check the time, then find themselves calculating how much sleep they can get if they fall asleep right away, as if sleep were some kind of timed exercise. That's not conducive to sleep! Still wearing a wristwatch? Leave it on the bureau where you can't reach or see it. And, if you've been using your phone for an alarm clock, it'll probably be better to get yourself a traditional alarm clock. Even if you have your phone on mute, it probably still flashes and can get your attention that way.

Sleep is for letting go of the outside world, and it will help to structure your bedroom accordingly.

Creating a Before-Bed Routine

How about getting ready for sleep? Here are a couple of guidelines. Disconnect from the Internet and your cell phone for at least thirty minutes before going to bed. Do something a little more traditional and low key, like reading (no murder mysteries!) or watching TV in another room. Pick a program that's not really engrossing or stimulating—talk shows are designed for this—and one that won't interfere with your scheduled bedtime.

Let go of the evening snacks. If you're sensitive to caffeine, limit any caffeinated beverages to early in the day. Go to bed at a time that will allow you to have the amount of sleep you think you need. Don't go to bed extra early hoping to increase your chances of getting enough sleep. That will likely ensure extra time of tossing and turning.

It would probably be good to spend a few minutes with a simple relaxation exercise before going to bed, or right upon getting into bed, like the belly breathing and meditation exercises in chapter 10. As with any relaxation technique, the key is to simply go through the steps and allow whatever happens to happen. Maybe you'll relax a little, maybe you'll relax a lot. Just take what comes your way. Don't strive to relax yourself!

Avoid napping during the day. When you sleep during the day, it often leads to less sleep at night, and you want to get back into the automatic habit of sleeping comfortably at night. So, even though it might seem like a good way to compensate for lost sleep, it probably just leads to more lost sleep. Get on a regular bedtime schedule and stick to it.

How soon will you or I fall asleep tonight? We just don't know exactly. The main point is to create the right conditions for sleep and allow whatever happens to happen.

Worry About Sleep is Just…Worry

Worry about sleep usually takes the form of this thought: *What if I don't get enough sleep?* The overwhelming majority of times, the answer to this question is that you will get sleepy. It's a self-correcting problem! It's not like the problem of, for example, dehydration. If I don't get enough water, I have to specifically correct that deficit; my body will not generate water on its own, and I have to find it and ingest it. When I get sleepy, my body will induce sleep. My main task with respect to sleep is to stay out of my own way and allow sleep to occur, rather than to make it occur.

Your best response to worries about troubled sleep will include handling worry about sleep separately from handling sleep. Handle worries about sleep the same way you handle any other comment from Uncle Argument. Treat it as worry, don't get fooled into taking the content very seriously, and humor the worries. Handle the activity of sleep in accordance with the sleep hygiene suggestions above.

What to do if you find it hard to fall asleep? Don't lie there for hours, trying to fall asleep. Give it a reasonable amount of time, perhaps half an hour. If you're unable to fall asleep within that time, I suggest you get up and engage in a brief period of activity.

What kind of activity? If you have a history of being able to relax yourself to sleep, perhaps with a book, then do that. But if you have a history of trying to relax yourself and failing, then don't do that again. Instead, take twenty minutes and work on some uncomfortable, boring chore, like scrubbing a floor or a bathtub. You just had the cleaning lady in today? Doesn't matter! The point of this task isn't to spruce up your place, it's to make sleep more inviting. If you get up and watch a TV show you like, or start a good book, it's likely to postpone sleep because you're doing something that's more interesting than sleep. Do a task that's less interesting for twenty minutes or so, then go back to bed. If you're still up in twenty or thirty minutes, repeat the process as needed.

Sometimes people fall into an unfortunate pattern of waking at the same time each night. It's usually a particularly unwanted time, like 2 a.m. This seems to occur because, after it happens once or twice, the person starts to worry—*What if I wake up at 2 a.m. again?*—and sure enough, like a self-fulfilling prophecy, they do. They get caught up in a vicious cycle of anticipatory worry about early wakening, followed by early wakening, followed by more worry, and on and on and on.

This is a classic example of chronic worry, in which worry about the possibility and uncertainty of early wakening leads to precisely the outcome you don't want. Here's a remedy I've found useful. It's not for the faint-hearted, because it has that classic aspect of medicine—helpful medicines always taste bad—but don't let that dissuade you.

When I work with clients who have this problem of habitual waking at 2 a.m., I usually suggest they set their alarm clock for 2. Then quickly, before they storm out of my office, I explain that it's the doubt and uncertainty about whether or not they will wake at 2 a.m. that feeds and breeds all the worry that actually wakes them, and creates the habitual early wakening. When they set the alarm in this manner, they no longer have any doubt about it. They're going to wake at 2 a.m.

This changes the problem. Before, they worried about whether or not they would wake up at 2 a.m. Now they know they will, and when they do, they can decide how to respond. Maybe they'll respond the same way they do every other time they wake early, but this is not what usually happens, and if it does, they're no worse off than before. What often does happen is that the person wakes in response to the alarm; wonders why the alarm has gone off; remembers that I asked them to set it that way; has a few choice thoughts for me, then turns it off and goes back to sleep. Sometimes people even find they wake a few minutes before the alarm, turn it off, and go back to sleep.

Even with this explanation, people often think it's a pretty weird idea, setting an alarm clock for 2 a.m. because they don't want to wake up at 2 a.m. And I guess it is. But this is a counterintuitive problem, and it requires a counterintuitive solution. When you need a counterintuitive solution, you can always turn to the Rule of Opposites. Setting the alarm for 2 a.m. is a pure application of the Rule of Opposites.

Worry on Awakening

Sometimes people experience the flip side of this problem. When they wake at the desired time in the morning, they lay in bed a while, trying to get a little more sleep. Instead of sleeping, though, they often juggle worrisome thoughts about their day as they lay there. Sometimes people even set their alarm a little earlier than they need, so they can build in an extra period of snoozing. The "snooze alarm" feature on some clocks encourages this practice.

Perhaps the best advice I can offer you about these "top of the morning" worries is this: don't take it lying down! You're at a big disadvantage as you lay there on your back, worrying, without anything else to do.

You'll be better off getting out of bed once you recognize that you are awake. Lying in bed, contemplating the bad things that might happen today, is not the way to start your day! Instead, get out of bed and start your morning routine—showering, having breakfast, letting the dog out. Get your day started, and postpone, for a short period, your contemplation of the day ahead.

After you've finished a portion of your morning routine, about fifteen minutes' worth, then sit down in a chair and take a few minutes to review the upcoming day. You'll be better able to view the day when you're fully awake and sitting up. If you "need" to worry in the morning, this is a better time and place to do it. If you have a strong habit of waking and worrying in bed, it might be a good alternative to schedule a worry appointment (chapter 10) as part of your morning routine.

Worries about Illness

Worry about possible disease and illness can be an especially challenging form of chronic worry.

Someone with "illness anxiety," as it's called by professionals, or someone who just has some tendencies in this regard, is going to experience lots of thoughts and concerns about the possibility that he has a disease. Sometimes this worry leads people to seek out much more medical attention than would otherwise seem necessary or desirable. Sometimes it leads people to do the opposite of that, to avoid ordinary medical checkups and procedures that would otherwise make good sense. We'll look at both responses here.

Too Much of a Good Thing

People who experience illness anxiety usually find themselves focused on some really serious and dread diseases, like cancer, Alzheimer's, AIDS, multiple sclerosis, heart ailments, and so on. You know what you're supposed to do if you detect a sign or symptom of some potential ailment, right? You go see the doctor and get it checked out! That makes sense.

The doctor should listen to your concern, examine the relevant parts of your body to evaluate it, and perhaps run some tests—blood work, X-rays, or other scans of relevant areas. In some cases, a consultation with a specialist may be part of the evaluation. The doctor's aim will be to clarify, to her satisfaction, whether or not an ailment exists; if so, to identify a course of treatment; and see any necessary treatment through to its successful conclusion.

But here's where it gets so tricky for people with chronic worry about the subject of a possible illness. If you have this kind of chronic worry, you arrive at the doctor's office with two goals in mind. First, you want the doctor's professional opinion as to whether or not you have a disease. If the doctor says you *do* have a disease, you want the doctor's recommendation for treatment. If the doctor says you *don't* have a disease, you want to be 100 percent confident that the doctor is correct—and that's a problem.

You Can't Always Get What You Want

No matter how healthy you may be, no matter how skilled, thorough, kind, and persuasive the doctor may be, you won't get the 100 percent certainty that you crave. Even if you feel that way during the visit, by the time you get home you'll probably start doubting all over again. This is the problem of trying to prove that something doesn't exist. It can't be done.

A person who worries a lot about her health may develop a concern about, say, having a dangerous heart condition, or stomach cancer. She'll notice physical sensations that seem to indicate that she has that disease—her heart occasionally changes speed or skips a beat, or her stomach produces sensations that she doesn't expect—and she'll consult a doctor about it.

She hopes to be able to prove that she doesn't have a disease and listens very closely to the words the doctor uses. If the doctor says, "I don't see any sign of this disease," she's unhappy with that, because it leaves open the possibility of the disease appearing in the future, maybe as soon as she leaves the office.

What she'd like the doctor to say is something more like, "You don't have this disease now, and I guarantee you will never get it in the future." That would sound good to her. But, it wouldn't be long before she'd start wondering, and get back to worrying. *How can the doctor be so sure?*

Doubting Your Doctor and Taking the Bait

What do you do when you find yourself once again worrying about the possibility that you have a dreaded disease and that the doctor, for whatever reason, failed to find it? If you're like most people with this concern, you respond to the doubt by engaging in a variety of anti-worry behaviors, just like the bull charges the red cape. You go back to that doctor to explain your situation again. You might have the thought that you left out an important detail the first time, or that you simply didn't emphasize it enough; or that the doctor overlooked it for some reason; or maybe even that the lab mislabeled your blood sample and you got someone else's report. So you go back and repeat the visit, asking the doctor to check again. You go to other doctors for other tests and opinions. You search the Internet. You ask friends and family for reassurance. But no matter how hard and thoroughly you try, there's Uncle Argument tapping you on the shoulder—"What if...?"

Wanting 100 Percent Certainty

It might seem to you as though this subject, a possible fatal illness, is too important to settle for less than 100 percent certainty. The fact is that no matter how important the subject seems, you can't have 100 percent certainty that a problem doesn't exist. The harder you try to attain it, the more painfully aware you will be that you're still not sure.

If this is your situation, you're not unsure because you failed to investigate your concern sufficiently. You're unsure because no one can be as sure as you wish. You've already attained your first goal, getting the doctor's opinion about your health. You're stuck trying to achieve your second goal—being 100 percent sure—and you're not going to achieve that goal.

You're not focused on this problem because undiagnosed disease is the biggest threat to your survival. It's not. There are any number of ordinary daily activities that carry more likelihood of death than undiagnosed disease, and you probably don't pay them much mind at all. You're stuck on this problem because it makes you feel so uncomfortable. It's discomfort, not danger. When you treat it like danger, the problem seems to spiral further out of control.

What can you do? The problem is that you're going to the doctor hoping to get a new opinion—from yourself. You're hoping to come home, thoroughly convinced and satisfied that you are healthy, without the disease that you feared, and that this certainty in your new opinion will last the rest of your life. But the only reason to go to the doctor is to get an opinion from the doctor, not to change your opinion or thoughts. You go there wanting to find out if the doctor thinks you have a disease. Make it your goal to get an opinion from the doctor, knowing that you will likely continue to have worrisome thoughts about disease before, during, and after your appointment. Don't go there for certainty, just go for the doctor's opinion.

Why Do I Do This to Myself?

Some people get stuck on this worry because they repeatedly have physical symptoms as well as worry. Anxiety is not all in your head. You will also experience it in your body. Some of the classic physical symptoms of anxiety include feeling lightheaded or dizzy; changes in your apparent heart rhythm or speed; muscular tightness in your chest, shoulders, back and neck; digestive distress; and more. Even though these are common symptoms of anxiety, some people who experience them have a lot of trouble accepting and believing that they can have physical symptoms that are just part of anxiety and not part of a physical disease.

People who worry about potential illnesses and find it hard to let go of those concerns frequently get angry at themselves. "I do it to myself!" they often say, and blame themselves for their troubles.

If you have worries about illness, and physical symptoms of anxiety as well, it's true that no one else is doing this to you. The worries and physical symptoms occur within your body and mind without outside cause, but this isn't really the same thing as you doing it to yourself. These worries and physical symptoms are natural, involuntary activity within your mind and body, part of the process by which we routinely scan and watch for signs of trouble.

If you have worries like these, you've got overzealous watch dogs! They bark when there's a prowler, and that's good. But they also bark when kids run across your lawn, or when the mailman leaves your mail. It's too much of a good thing! But they are dogs, after all, and it's probably unhelpful to expect that they only bark when there's an actual threat and never bark when there isn't. They're not doing it to bother you; they're doing it because that's their nature.

In the same way, it's within all of us to watch for signs of possible trouble and seek to head it off. That's a part of our nature, and sometimes we get more of it than we might wish. That's a problem. But it's not your fault.

Avoiding a Good Thing

Other people will respond to chronic worry about possible illness in a very different fashion. They avoid doctor visits like the plague. People who get caught up in this pattern go for years without seeing a doctor. They avoid annual physicals as well as the usual recommended milestones, like colonoscopies at certain intervals after age fifty, a shingles vaccination at age sixty, and so on. The necessity of a medical visit, perhaps for a chest X-ray required by a new employer, or for an actual medical emergency, often becomes a crisis for people with this kind of worry. If you're someone with this kind of experience, your worries take a different form compared to people who constantly seek out medical evaluations.

Why does illness anxiety lead people to avoid doctors? There are several reasons.

One common pattern is that people worry not about the potential effects of a disease, but rather about the shock and anxiety they think they'll feel if a doctor tells them of one. If you have this type of chronic worry, your chief concern is an imagined, hypothetical moment when the doctor examines you, or reads your lab report, looks up at you with a heavy sigh, and says, "I have bad news."

People with this form of illness anxiety imagine this scenario frequently, and the thought of hearing bad news scares them so much they think they have to avoid that possibility at all costs. It's similar to the anticipatory fear a person with panic disorder feels when they imagine getting into a situation they associate with panic attacks, perhaps an airplane or crowded elevator.

White-Coat Syndrome

A routine part of most doctor visits is a blood pressure reading. Some people hate and fear this to such an extent that it leads them to avoid the doctor. Maybe they have a pattern, called "white coat syndrome," in which their blood pressure goes up when it's time for the reading, and they have such an anticipatory reaction to this that they get caught up in a vicious cycle. They imagine the nurse saying something like, "Oh my God, your blood pressure is through the roof!" and causing a scene, while their blood pressure continues to mount.

People who experience anticipatory worry about the blood pressure reading, the doctor's feedback, or any other aspect of the office visit sometimes find it intolerable to wait their turn in the waiting room, because that's prime time for anticipatory "what if" thoughts to arise. Just like the fearful flier who gets to the gate only to turn back, sometimes people get as far as the waiting room only to leave in response to heightened anticipatory fears.

Worry About Illness Is Just...Worry

If you recognize yourself in the above descriptions, and see that chronic worry about health and illness is having a negative effect on your life, then the fact that the apparent content of the worry is about health and illness becomes much less important. Think back to chapter 6, in which we diagrammed the typical worry sentence. The content of the worry sentence is revealed to be of very little importance when we consider the meaning of the "what if" clause that precedes it. Do you remember what the "what if" part means?

It means "let's pretend." Whatever follows that pretend clause—cancer or the common cold—it's still pretend! You're still multiplying by zero!

That's what you end up with when "what if" thoughts get you to pretend, even about topics that would be very important outside of pretending.

Don't Hide Your Worry!

It's very common for people who struggle with chronic worry about illness to try to deny and hide it when they visit the doctor. Do you do this? Some of this is motivated by a desire to not be hampered by this problem—you probably don't want to "give in to it." Some of it is from embarrassment. It's also often motivated by a concern that, if you acknowledge to the doctor that you have some trouble with worry, all your medical concerns and complaints will be dismissed as simply "anxiety related."

These are understandable concerns. However, to the extent that they lead you to disguise or deny your troubles with worry, they probably make your situation more difficult rather than better. If you have chronic worry about illness, you really have two problems to bring to the doctor: the symptoms you want to investigate, and your burning desire to prove, beyond a shadow of doubt, that you are not ill. If you only acknowledge the symptoms, without acknowledging how your quest for certainty complicates your life, then both you and the doctor may get diverted into unproductive areas.

Some physicians, seeing that the patient is not entirely satisfied with the diagnosis of good health, will suggest test after test and specialist after specialist, either not noticing that chronic worry is part of the issue or preferring to avoid dealing with it. You can waste a lot of time and money this way! You will also probably be disappointed to find that no amount of tests and consultations will give you the perfect reassurance you seek. In fact, the more tests you have, the more opportunities for worry will come your way.

Your internal process of worry continues to go forward whether you acknowledge it or not. If worry about possible illness is part of your lot in life, hiding that from your physician may well make the doctor-patient relationship seem more adversarial and less helpful. However, if you can acknowledge and discuss with your physician the way worry influences your thinking about your health, you may find it easier to arrive at a more satisfying working relationship with that doctor.

Some physicians probably don't want any part of this and would prefer to have obedient, cooperative patients who accept their recommendations and don't worry about it. If you happen to have such a physician, you may well need to change doctors and find one who is more open to working around the way worry influences your medical treatment.

Thinking It Over

Worries about sleep and health follow the general pattern of all chronic worry, and may also lead to the creation of strong habits that increase and maintain your worry. This chapter identified some characteristic behaviors that people adopt hoping to get the worry under their control, behaviors which ultimately make the worry more persistent and severe rather than less. Identifying such behaviors, and reversing them, is an important part of changing your relationship with chronic worry.

CHAPTER 14

Closing Thoughts: There's Something Funny About Worry...

So there you have it. Chronic worry is not an intruder or a disease you have to oppose. It's a bunch of reactions that appear in your internal world, in your mind, when you try too hard to control and oppose unwanted worrisome thoughts. Chronic worry tricks you into taking it seriously and opposing it just like a matador tricks a bull into charging men armed with swords and spikes.

A matador tricks a bull with a red cape. Chronic worry tricks you with a phrase like "What if...?"

When you fall for the trick, you end up arguing with Uncle Argument and feeling nauseous at a banquet that you had hoped to enjoy. And the best way to defuse the situation with Uncle Argument is to playfully humor him.

This might not be as hard as it seems, because there's something funny about worry.

I give frequent workshops on worry and anxiety at professional mental health conferences around the country. These are usually held in large hotels or conference facilities with rooms for many workshops to occur simultaneously. At break times, as participants from other meetings walk by my table, they often have an interesting reaction. When people see the sign for the meeting about worry, they frequently laugh and say something like this: "Oh, I could really use this meeting!"

Nobody seems to do that at the tables for meetings on depression, schizophrenia, eating disorders, and so on. There's something funny about worry. We can recognize it if we're open to it, and it helps change our relationship with worry when we do.

Responding to chronic worry without humor is like drilling a tooth without local anesthesia. You can do it if you have to, but it's so much easier, and more comfortable, with humor.

I remember a client who came to see me in her late thirties, seeking help with a severe illness anxiety. This is a condition in which people are extremely fearful of terrible diseases, so much so that they're always looking for signs of illness and often fearing they've found some, when they're not actually ill. During our first meeting, she told me, "All my life I've been afraid I'll die young."

I pointed out that it was probably too late, that the earliest she could die now would be middle-aged. After she got over the urge to slap me, she laughed really hard, and talked about all the worries she'd experienced that never came close to happening. Putting the funny part of her worry on the table like that helped her get some emotional distance from the upset she'd been feeling, and helped her tackle the worry trick more directly.

Another client comes to mind who sought help with panic attacks. She frequently had panic attacks in situations where she could be observed by others, like waiting rooms and grocery stores. She didn't fear that the panic attack would harm her, but that it would make her look "like a crazy person" and scare everyone around her. Chief among her fears was the idea that her eyes would bug out and her hair would stand up.

We could have spent a lot of time talking about the kinetic properties of hair, and whether or not this was possible, but it seemed like a waste of time, akin to arguing about your worries. Instead, I asked her to take some observations next time she had a panic attack, and she was agreeable. I asked her to keep a six-inch ruler and a compact mirror with her at all times, and in the event of a panic attack she was to measure how high her hair stood.

She had a panic attack several days later, in the waiting room of her physician. She raced out of there and headed for the lobby, then remembered that she had to measure her hair. She detoured into the bathroom, planted herself in front of a mirror, and pulled her yellow ruler out of her purse. She held it up to her scalp and gazed into the mirror. There she was, holding a yellow ruler to her head, and she just burst out laughing on seeing this! That was pretty much the end of hair standing up.

That's an example of "humoring the fear." It involves accepting the fear rather than arguing with it, and confronting the situation as concretely as possible. This often helps the funny part of the fear to emerge and can be much more powerful than logically and rationally trying to debate and change your thoughts.

I've previously mentioned that I have some humorous songs on my website. Here's an excerpt from another one, the first verse of a song sung to the tune of "Folsom Prison" (apologies to Johnny Cash).

I feel my heart start racing
That's when I hold my breath
It makes me feel light headed and
I start thinking of death
Oh, I think I will go crazy
And that my heart will burst.
Now they say that's never happened,
Hah! I bet I'll be the first!

Visitors to my website love these songs. What makes the songs so funny? The lyrics above simply depict the typical thoughts of a person having a bad panic attack. I didn't add a separate joke or punchline, yet people who struggle with panic attacks and regularly have the thoughts in these lyrics hear this song and have a good belly laugh. Hearing the thoughts in a song just makes it easier for them to find the funny part, the trick, and to step away from their more usual reaction of disgust and despair.

Freud had some interesting observations about humor. He suggested at one point that humor served the purpose of saving various kinds of "mental energy" and releasing them. He described "savings in mental energy" devoted to anger and fear when the individual suddenly realizes that what appeared to be dangerous isn't dangerous at all. He also cited a release of mental energy devoted to thinking when the individual suddenly realizes that all that thinking is actually unnecessary. It's the energy that was previously locked up in unnecessary overthinking and fight-or-flight responses that drives the laughter and humorous response.[1]

I think that's exactly what happened with my client as she gazed at herself, and her yellow ruler, in the mirror. All that overthinking, and fight-or-flight response, was suddenly revealed as a misunderstanding, and she laughed.

Perhaps you've already had the experience of laughing at some question or experiment I've suggested earlier in the book. It's good if you have! There's something funny about worry, and if you can get in touch with that funny part, it will probably be pretty helpful for you in changing your relationship with worry.

I hasten to add that this works only so long as it's the individual experiencing the worry who finds the funny part humorous. So, friends and family of chronic worriers—don't take this as license to take the lead and start making jokes about their worrying!

So that's the book. I hope you found it helpful, and I hope you will continue to find it helpful in guiding your path to a different—and better—relationship with the worry that is a part of everyone's life.

Notes

Chapter 4

1. Pittman, Catherine, and Elizabeth Karle. 2009. *Extinguishing Anxiety*. South Bend, Indiana: Foliadeux Press.

Chapter 5

1. Baer, Lee. 2001. *The Imp of the Mind*. New York: The Penguin Group.

2. Hayes, Steven, Kirk Strosahl, and Kelly Wilson. 1999. *Acceptance and Commitment Therapy*. New York: The Guilford Press.

3. Hayes, Strosahl, and Wilson. 1999.

4. Weekes, Claire. 1962. *Hope and Help for Your Nerves*. New York: Penguin Books.

Chapter 7

1. Wegner, Daniel. 1989. *White Bears and Other Unwanted Thoughts*. New York: Viking Penguin.

2. Quoted in Luoma, Jason, Steven Hayes, and Robyn Walser. 2007. *Learning ACT*. Oakland, CA: New Harbinger Publications. 57.

3. Hayes, Steven, Kirk Strosahl, and Kelly Wilson. 1999. *Acceptance and Commitment Therapy*. New York: The Guilford Press.

Chapter 14

1. Freud, Sigmund. 1905/1990. *Jokes and Their Relation to the Unconscious*. New York: Norton.

David A. Carbonell, PhD, is a clinical psychologist who specializes in the treatment of anxiety disorders in Chicago, IL. He is the "coach" at *www.anxietycoach.com*, and author of *Panic Attacks Workbook*.

Foreword writer **Sally M. Winston, PsyD,** founded and directed the anxiety disorders treatment program at The Sheppard and Enoch Pratt Hospital in Baltimore, MD. She served as the first chair of the Clinical Advisory Board of the Anxiety and Depression Association of America (ADAA), and received their inaugural Jerilyn Ross Clinician Advocate Award. She is coauthor of *What Every Therapist Needs to Know About Anxiety Disorders.*

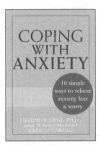
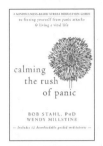
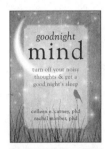
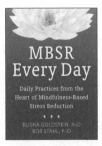
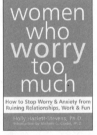
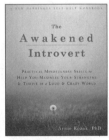

Register your **new harbinger** titles for additional benefits!

When you register your **new harbinger** title—purchased in any format, from any source—you get access to benefits like the following:

- Downloadable accessories like printable worksheets and extra content

- Instructional videos and audio files

- Information about updates, corrections, and new editions

Not every title has accessories, but we're adding new material all the time.

Access free accessories in 3 easy steps:

1. Sign in at NewHarbinger.com (or **register** to create an account).

2. Click on **register a book**. Search for your title and click the **register** button when it appears.

3. Click on the **book cover or title** to go to its details page. Click on **accessories** to view and access files.

That's all there is to it!

If you need help, visit:

NewHarbinger.com/accessories

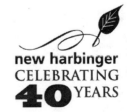
new harbinger
CELEBRATING
40 YEARS